EASY PREGNANCY W

EASY PREGNANCY WITH YOGA

STELLA WELLER

Illustrated by Jane Bowden

THORSONS PUBLISHING GROUP

First published in the United Kingdom 1979
This revised and expanded edition published 1991

British Library Cataloguing in Publication Data

Weller, Stella
  Easy pregnancy with yoga.
  Rev. ed
  1. Pregnant women. Physical fitness. Hatha — yoga
  I. Title
  613.7046

ISBN 0-7225-1931-1

Published by Thorsons Publishers Limited,
Wellingborough, Northamptonshire NN8 2RQ, England

Typeset by Harper Phototypesetters Limited,
Northampton, England
Printed in Great Britain by The Bath Press, Bath, Avon

10 9 8 7 6 5 4 3 2 1

Acknowledgements

I thank all who have helped me with this book through their good wishes and encouragement.

I am especially grateful to my husband, Walter, and my sons, Karl and David, for their patience while I did research and wrote the script for this book.

I am particularly grateful, too, to Dr O. H. Webber for reading and evaluating the script and for writing the foreword.

Many thanks to Dr C. W. Simpson for his suggestions for the chapter on caesarean birth.

Special thanks to Iris Weverman, Reg.Pht., Childbirth Educator, for her important suggestions for the post partum section.

Finally, I wish to express much appreciation to all at Thorsons for their reliability and courtesy. Special thanks go to John Hardaker, and the editorial staff; and Judith Smallwood and staff in the Publicity and Promotions Department.

Contents

Foreword

In my 25 years of medical practice I have seen a marked change in the process of childbirth. So-called 'natural childbirth' is, I think, much closer to reality than it once was. The main change that seems to explain this is the increased knowledge of the new mother (and her partner) obtained through prenatal classes. Here the prospective parents are prepared for the process and trained in the necessary exercises and breathing techniques. It is these learned skills that seem to have made the difference, allowing the new mother, often with her partner's help, to deliver her child confidently and naturally.

Mrs Weller's book is something I welcome in my practice as a guide for these exercise and breathing routines during pregnancy and delivery. It integrates the now popular yoga techniques with the necessary exercise and breathing techniques of pregnancy and delivery. I think it is well worth reading and following her regimen.

O. H. Webber, MD

Introduction

The purpose of this book is primarily to provide pregnant women with a selection of easily adaptable bodily movements, positions, and breathing techniques which they can use for conditioning throughout pregnancy. Any woman, however, who wishes to improve herself will find this information most helpful.

Childbirth preparation classes usually offer, among other things, the opportunity for conditioning the body in preparation of labour, but this preparation lasts only for about eight to ten weeks. I believe that a woman could condition her entire organism in a much sounder way if such conditioning were to cover a longer period of time, and be carried out in a gentler, more gradual way. She could do this by each day using techniques such as are described in this book. If she applies them faithfully to her own specific needs, not only would she be preparing herself for actively participating in the birth of her baby, but she would also be consciously promoting a more comfortable, healthier pregnancy in which there would be a minimum of discomfort and a maximum of vital energy.

If you are pregnant, do attend childbirth preparation classes. There you will meet other women who are having an experience similar to yours. You will have a chance to share with them some of your hopes and fears, and discuss the various phenomena of pregnancy. You will be reassured and gain a better perspective of your situation when you discover that they also are going through many of the things you yourself are experiencing. And you will have the benefit of the personal help and guidance of trained teachers. Classes also offer your husband a chance to become further involved with your pregnancy, and allow him to better understand the ways in which you may be reacting to the many changes which are taking place in your body.

Exercise is only one aspect of prenatal care. As part of your preparation for what should be one of the most exciting events of your life, you should establish a good rapport with your doctor. Since he/she will be the one best acquainted with the course of your pregnancy, his/her instructions should always take predominance over all other considerations. Ask your doctor as many questions as you feel you need in order to enlighten yourself as fully as possible.

There are also many excellent and authoritative books dealing with pregnancy and childbirth at libraries and bookstores. Please make use of them, but use them wisely. Encourage your husband to read at least one of them, so as to increase his understanding of pregnancy and better equip him to give you the emotional support which is so vital to you at this time.

You will notice that there are several repetitions in this book. They are intentional, and are meant as reminders, as a form of constant encouragement, and for ease of reference.

I realize that there are many women who do not care to set aside a specific number of minutes daily for prescribed exercises. If you are one of them, you can incorporate some of the poses, breathing and relaxation techniques, and other comfort measures into your usual dialy routine. Fit them wherever practicable into your household and other duties. These exercises can be fun when used in this way, and suggestions for doing so are given in the text.

Pregnancy is not an illness but a natural function. Although there was a time when a pregnant woman was thought to be in a 'delicate state' and encouraged to do as little as possible, pregnancy is now considered a time when a woman should be at her fittest so as to meet the increased demands made of her not only physically, but also mentally and emotionally. Because of these added demands at this time, the dividing line between good health and illness is finer than during the non-pregnant state.

The human body is so constructed that in order to remain healthy it must be exercised regularly and correctly. There is no doubt that suitable exercise performed daily throughout pregnancy will help to produce and maintain good general muscle tone and, in particular, strengthen and keep in a healthy, elastic condition those muscles which will be used especially during childbirth. Housework, however abundant, is not in itself a satisfactory enough form of exercise since it brings into play only some muscles while others, notably those of the pelvic floor which are the ones most involved in the process of childbirth, are usually neglected altogether. In many cases housework is just the type of activity which causes fatigue. A suitable regimen of appropriate exercises, however, such as yoga provides, promotes relaxation at its best. The results which yoga can produce are in strong contrast with the many side effects often associated with household duties: irritability, depression and general fatigue.

It is generally accepted that a woman can better approach childbirth with calm and confidence if her muscles are in good tone and she has learned how to control them; if she has understood breath control; if she has taught herself how to relax completely at will, and if she has taken nutritional and other

measures to maintain good general health. Postnatally, the woman who has followed a regimen of suitable exercise, coupled with correct breathing during her pregnancy will find that, as she continues her exercises she very quickly recovers her strength (providing that everything has followed a normal course). She speedily regains her figure and in some cases acquires a better one, and is able to enjoy her family and life in general, more fully.

The yoga system of physical exercise is ideal for the pregnant woman. It calls for very gentle, rhythmic movements, and emphasizes that one should never strain or push oneself beyond one's comfortable limit. It stresses proper breathing, and draws attention to the many benefits of complete relaxation.

The word 'yoga' comes from the Sanskrit 'yuj' meaning 'yoke' or 'joining together'. It has many interpretations. Yoga asanas (postures), by strengthening and disciplining the physical body, automatically bring clarity to the mind and stability to the emotions. The overall result is a joining together of healthy body, alert mind and stable emotions into a well-integrated, self-confident individual. This is but one interpretation. Yoga postures are many thousands of years old and are based on sound anatomical and physiological principles which are in agreement with medical and scientific knowledge of the West.

As mentioned earlier, the postures are designed to tone and strengthen not only the skeletal muscles, but the glands and organs of the body, thereby generally improving the blood circulation and the functioning of the entire organism. This is why yoga is so suitable for the pregnant woman; no strain whatever is involved if correctly applied, and fatigue is not allowed to accumulate.

Within recent years there has been growing appreciation and acceptance in medical and related circles of the interdependence of body, mind and emotions. Yoga postures benefit all these simultaneously, promoting physical fitness, sound nerves and a calmer personality. The influence of the mind and emotions on childbirth is profound, as many doctors and scientists will attest.

When I was studying obstetrics, we, the students, were required to perform prenatal exercises and breathing patterns based on the psycholoprophylaxis method of childbirth preparation. Participating in these exercises provided us with better insight, understanding and patience to help women in labour. Later, when I began to practise Hatha Yoga (physical yoga) I was amazed at the similarity between many of the asanas (postures) and the prenatal exercises we had learned. I subsequently discovered that some authorities claim that the psychoprophylaxis techniques are largely based on yoga which is many thousands of years old. It appeared to me that the yoga method was, in actual fact, ideal for the pregnant woman. It is gentle, rhythmic, non-fatiguing, working not only on muscles to improve their tone, but also on the nervous system, and through the breath to stabilize the emotions. In short, yoga seemed to me to meet more fully the needs of the pregnant woman, whether these needs be physical, mental or emotional.

During pregnancy the body is subject to many additional stresses and strains — larger volume of circulating blood, harder work for the heart, greater weight for the skeletal and other muscles to support, a greater tendency to emotional upsets, and more susceptibility to tension and therefore fatigue. It is thus essential, not only to the welfare of the woman but also to that of the unborn child, that the body be kept superbly fit and beautifully relaxed. The woman should learn how to conserve energy and forestall fatigue before it accumulates to any significant degree. How indispensable and how very welcome are good muscle tone, a plentiful reserve of energy, a calm attitude, the ability to relax adequately at will, and the capacity to cooperate fully with obstetrical attendants as they instruct you in suitable breathing and other comfort measures during labour! Yoga can help you achieve all this.

Make the most of your pregnancy. It can be a very fruitful time — a time for character building, and a time for cultivating healthful habits which can be of tremendous benefit, not only to you, but through you to your family. I do hope that my book will in some small way contribute to your health, comfort and well-being during this most privileged time.

S.A.W.

Chapter 1

Instructions and Cautions for Practising the Asanas (Postures)

Before attempting any of the postures or breathing techniques described in this book, be sure to *check with your doctor* and obtain permission to practise them. If you have a history of actual or threatened miscarriage, you would be wise not to do them in the first three or four months of pregnancy. If your pregnancy is following a normal course, you may use all or most of the techniques described herein. Adapt them to suit your body and omit any at the first sign of discomfort as you become larger.

If you have engaged actively in some form of exercise on a regular basis, and have kept fit prior to becoming pregnant, you will be able to perform the postures more readily than a woman who has not done so. If you are attempting a regular exercise programme for the first time, it would be wise to start with the simpler movements, and perform these with the utmost care so as to give the body time to get used to what may be considered a new experience. Do not expect to make up overnight for years of lack of regular exercise. Also, you may find yoga postures so enjoyable that you may become too enthusiastic and want to practise them more than you should. You must not do this.

Yoga does not provide the key to a painless childbirth. It can, however, help make the experience much easier, and will certainly contribute to a more comfortable pregnancy, if used regularly but moderately.

When you first start to do the asanas, keep your exercise periods very short. If for some reason you must discontinue exercise for one or more days, start again gradually, doing such things as the Sponge (section 6), any of the easier poses, and the breathing exercises.

When to practise

Choose a convenient time for your exercise session, and if possible, try to practise at the same time each day. Before breakfast is best, since the stomach is empty. However, if you are experiencing morning sickness it would be wise to postpone exercise until later in the day, doing only some breathing exercises and the Sponge on arising. Although the body is somewhat stiff at this time, regular exercise will conquer this. Beginning your day with exercises will give you much needed energy and will help you work more efficiently. Practising in the evening can help eliminate fatigue accumulated during the day and induce sound sleep. Some people, however, find that exercising in the evening is too stimulating. Some of you may find it more suitable to divide practice time into two or more periods of shorter duration. You may perhaps do some breathing exercises and gentle limbering up on arising, and the postures before lunch and/or supper.

Practise daily. It is much better to practise for only ten minutes each day than for half an hour twice a week. Start with about five or ten minutes daily, working up to about a total of twenty minutes. Generally speaking, I believe that more than this at any one time may be too much. You want to avoid monotony and, at all costs, fatigue.

Food

Whatever time best suits you, make sure that two or three hours have elapsed since you last ate (depending on the size and content of the meal), and try not to eat for about half an hour after practising, if possible.

Hygiene

Ideally the bladder should be empty and the bowel evacuated before exercising. If you are especially stiff, you may find that a warm bath taken before practising helps you move more easily. A hot bath is best avoided as it will rob you of much needed energy. Do not take a bath for at least twenty minutes following exercise.

Where to practise

Choose a quiet, darkened room. Air it out first and, depending on the weather, leave a window open or closed, but avoid draughts. Try to have no interruptions while exercising, as concentration is of great importance to the effectiveness of the asanas. Wherever possible, you may practise in your garden or other convenient place out of doors. Spread a mat or a couple of folded blankets on the ground. The surface on which you practise should be firm, even and comfortable.

Remove from your person any object which may hurt you or cause pressure — hair ornaments, glasses, belt, ring, etc., and make sure that your clothing is loose, light, and very comfortable.

Limbering up

Before proceeding with specific asanas you should always do a few limbering-up movements. This will increase your body temperature slightly, making it easier for you to move your joints. The exercises will give a gentle stretch to muscles and ligaments and increase blood circulation. By gently warming up your body in this way you will not risk joint or muscle strain. Dancers usually perform limbering-up exercises before going into the actual dance, and pianists play scales and other finger exercises before they attempt a serious piece of music. In the same way, you should engage in limbering up your body before practising the postures.

Several such exercises appear to me to be especially suitable for the pregnant woman; these are listed on pages 79-81.

How to practise

First, spend a few minutes in complete relaxation. The Sponge (section 6) is recommended. Follow this with some limbering-up movements (section 1) to prepare the body for the poses. When ready for the postures, perform them gently, smoothly and rhythmically at all times. There must never be the slightest strain or attempt to go beyond your particular bodily limitation. With patience and perseverance the movements will become increasingly easy to do. *The attempt is really what matters most and not the completed posture.*

Before attempting a posture, visualize it completely in your mind; keep this image before you as a goal toward which to strive. Go into a posture slowly and with control, combining effortless breathing with the movements specified for that posture. Breathing properly during the exercises provides the muscles with an adequate supply of oxygen to help them work effectively and to combat a build up of the substances which cause fatigue. When you have gone as far as comfort permits, hold the position for one, two, or more seconds *without* holding the breath; breathe as normally as possible during this holding period.

Slowly come out of the position, again incorporating the right breathing. Finally you relax. Always rest briefly between postures and for about ten minutes at the very end of your exercise session. At this time you should practise the Sponge. Your body will have a chance to absorb vital energy and eliminate fatigue poisons.

After childbirth

Again *check with your doctor* before doing any form of exercise. He or she is the one most familiar with the nature of your labour and subsequent progress. You may also have had an episiotomy (incision of the pelvic floor to facilitate birth) which will need time to heal. If you are permitted to exercise, start with the lighter postures, the breathing exercises and, of course, the Sponge (section 6).

Chapter 2

The Sitting Postures

The benefits of the sitting postures are many. Because we are used to sitting on chairs from an early age, our ankle, knee, and hip joints become inflexible sooner than those of people who are used to sitting in the positions described in this chapter. Try to spend part of each day in one of these sitting attitudes. It does not matter if you sit on the floor, on a sofa, or some other suitable furniture. If you have never practised any of these postures you will experience some difficulty at first in trying to get into them though they appear simple. Do not be discouraged. As your ligaments stretch and joints become more supple, you will be amazed at the ease with which you will be able to adopt these postures. At first you may try placing a large cushion or pillow on top of the rug or folded blankets on which you do your exercises. You will find it easier to do the sitting positions by sitting on this cushion or pillow. As soon as your back begins to feel the slightest fatigue, give it support by shifting yourself against the wall or other available prop (still sitting on your cushion or pillow). Suitable aids for supporting the back are pillows or cushions. Spend only a minute or two in the sitting posture of your choice, gradually increasing the length of time you sit in this manner as you become more limber. Use your hands to help you into and out of position whenever necessary.

As preparation for practising the sitting postures, I suggest the Leg Flop (section 1).

The postures listed in section 2 will give you a firm and stable base on which to rest the body while sitting. They will hold your spine naturally erect so that all your internal organs will fall into their intended positions and not be cramped. These postures will contribute to the unimpeded circulation of blood to the internal organs, with resulting improvement in their functioning. Since posture is generally improved when in these positions, you will find it easier to breathe more deeply and more efficiently, so that your body and that of the child within you will be better oxygenated. Because your breathing is improved your mind will be clearer and your emotions more stable. The sitting postures strengthen the back and abdomen as well as loosen the ankle, knee and hip joints. All the cross-legged poses stretch, tone, and strengthen the adductor muscles which run along the inner thighs and so contribute to the health of the pelvic floor. By making the muscles of the pelvic floor strong and elastic, the cross-legged positions help to facilitate the birth of the baby. Finally, since the pelvic floor muscles are the main supports of the uterus, bladder, and other pelvic organs, strengthening them will help prevent prolapse of these organs in later life.

Only a few of the simpler sitting postures will be described. Even those who have never exercised before on a regular basis should be able to do them. Try to remember that the benefits of these postures are so many that perseverance is worthwhile.

Caution

Because the sitting postures (with one exception) exert a certain amount of pressure on the legs and temporarily slow down the blood circulation in these parts, they ought not to be practised by those who have varicose veins. Such persons can, however, do the dynamic variation of the Squatting Pose (p.87) and the Sitting Warrior (p.86) in both static and dynamic forms.

Suggestions for fitting the sitting postures into the daily routine

Use the cross-legged positions (Easy Pose and Perfect Posture) when sewing, knitting, reading, watching television, mixing a cake by hand, chatting, doing breathing exercises, meditating, etc. The Disciple Posture can also be used in this way. The Firm Posture may be adopted for any of the foregoing activities, and if you curl the toes forward rather than have them pointing straight backward, you may care to experiment with having tea or a snack at a low table in this position, Japanese style.

The ways in which you can fit squatting into your daily routine are innumerable. Here are a few examples. Squat with your legs in broad stance when about to pick up a fallen object, attend to a small child or chat casually with someone (primitive people are seldom seen to stand and chat; they squat instead, one reason why they do not as a rule suffer from the many back disorders we 'civilized' people do. They stand mainly in preparation for moving from one place to another!). Squat to dust lower parts of furniture, tie shoelaces, polish shoes or silverware, tidy low cupboards, take something from a low drawer, fold laundry, do gardening, etc.

Be constantly on the lookout for ways in which to incorporate these and other postures into your everyday activities; it can be fun and will certainly be rewarding.

Chapter 3

Strengthening the Back and Abdomen

The back, which is normally subjected to a great deal of strain, is more heavily taxed during pregnancy. If the strength and suppleness of the back were to be maintained by means of suitable and regular exercise, common conditions such as drooping shoulders, arched back, sunken chest, sagging breasts, and an unduly exaggerated inward curve of the lower spine could be avoided, with consequent improvement of posture. With this improvement of posture would come stronger back and abdominal muscles, stronger pelvic floor muscles, and a drastic reduction of minor aches and pains, especially in the lower back. The internal organs would fall into their correct anatomical positions, and the entire body would function more healthfully.

What is essentially desirable in the abdomen is to achieve good tone and strength of the muscles. By strength I do not mean that these muscles should be made hard and rigid through exercise, but that their ability to contract and relax efficiently should be improved. Strengthening the abdominal muscles would be yet another contribution to minimal pain during labour.

When you consider the vital organs which are contained within the abdominal cavity, and the nature of the work performed by them — digestion of food, circulation of blood, elimination of waste matter and so on — you will perhaps better appreciate the importance of keeping the trunk firm and healthy. The health of the trunk and the organs it contains cannot be achieved without due consideration to the muscles which are very much a part of their formation. Good posture is an integral part of the health of the abdominal muscles. If the muscles are lax posture will be poor, and vice versa. The internal organs will suffer by being cramped.

If the muscles are weak, postnatal recovery will be slower with accompanying poor tone and elasticity, and the abdomen will sag and be unsightly. Posture will be affected, the back will be subjected to undue stress, the internal organs will suffer, and a whole vicious cycle will begin. Care must be taken to keep the muscles healthy, partly through regular exercise.

The muscles of the back and those of the abdomen complement each other. When those of the back are contracted those of the abdomen are stretched and vice versa. The following asanas have therefore been chosen because they involve both sets of muscles and are simple to perform. They have also been selected because they are effective in toning, strengthening and improving the elasticity of these muscles.

During pregnancy, the body's centre of gravity is altered by the increase in size and weight of the uterus. The result is that the pelvis is tilted in such a way as to increase the lumbar curve of the spine. With this increased spinal curvature often comes back strain and backache. However, strengthening the abdominal muscles and those of the back, as well as observing correct postural habits, can control these abnormal conditions and keep them to a minimum.

During the expulsive stage of labour when

the baby is being literally pushed out of the birth canal, good abdominal muscle tone will be an asset, as it will enable you to contribute more actively to the pushing action that will help your baby to be born.

Caution

In persons not accustomed to regular exercise, the abdominal muscles are often weak. For this reason it would be wise to start doing movements involving these muscles very slowly and carefully. The muscles will, with regular exercise, gradually acquire strength and elasticity.

The Raised Leg Posture (section 1) is a suitable warm-up in preparation for the asanas which follow. Another effective limbering-up technique is the Cat Pose (which is also an asana). When performed as a pose, follow the usual practice of going into position slowly, holding, and then coming out of position equally slowly. As a warm-up exercise, follow one movement by the other in a smooth, undulating motion.

Chapter 4

Posture and Body Mechanics

As the uterus increases in size and weight during pregnancy, the body's centre of gravity shifts in order to maintain balance. This change accounts for the increased curvature of the lower back which is to be expected, to some extent. However, if abdominal muscle tone is poor, the abdomen will protrude quite markedly rather than enlarge upward and thus cause the pelvis to tilt forward much more than it should. The results are greater strain on the sacroiliac joints at the back of the pelvis, an exaggerated curve of the lower spine, and harmful stress on all the muscles and ligaments which support the spine. Together, these abnormal conditions lead to excessive fatigue. And we know that on no account should a woman become overtired during pregnancy.

When the body is properly aligned and habits of good posture are practised, the internal organs fall naturally into their intended positions and function well. When, however, one indulges in faulty habits of holding and moving the body, the internal organs are subjected to undesirable pressures, and the blood circulation is impeded. In short, these organs can no longer function as efficiently as they should, and many distressing physical and mental conditions can and do result. Often, one does not suspect that symptoms such as constipation, digestive disorders, backache, headache, shortness of breath, cold hands and feet, and depression can be related to habitual bad posture; but they can. Indeed, reliable accounts verify that many people who for years have suffered from the complaints just mentioned, and yet others who have had disorders of the lungs, heart and pelvic organs, have been greatly relieved and even cured by cultivating habits of good posture and body mechanics.

Good body alignment and correct postural habits whenever sitting or standing, lying down or getting up, will contribute to a feeling of well-being, to good overall muscle tone, and above all, to the reduction of tension and fatigue. Habitual good posture will contribute to the strength and health of the pelvic floor and will give a measure of relief from pressure on the bladder. Correct posture is well worth cultivating, not only because of its great contribution to comfort during pregnancy, but indeed as an indispensable asset throughout life.

Sitting

The sitting postures and the squatting position have already been described (chapter 2, section 2), and should be practised for a portion of each day. Since, however, we in the West, for the most part, are used to sitting on chairs from childhood, we cannot suddenly be expected to squat or sit cross-legged on the floor for long periods daily. Many of us, however, sit incorrectly, and apart from appearing sloppy, this habit can and often does result in backache. Figure 1 is an example of a *poor* sitting posture. You need not sit rigidly to sit correctly. Here is one comfortable yet sound way of sitting:

1. Sit as far back on a chair as will allow the small of your back to touch the back of it for support. Make sure you are sitting on your 'sitting bones' (you may be able to feel them with your hands, one under each buttock) and not on the tail bone which is at the bottom of the spine.

2. Place your feet on a footstool, hassock, or other suitable piece of furniture, so that the knees are bent and are higher than the hips (Fig. 2. A stool has been used instead of a chair to give a clearer view of the alignment of the body). In this position the curve of the spine at the small of the back is considerably reduced, thereby relieving pressure on the discs between the bones which make up the spine. This in turn contributes markedly to a reduction of strain on the back with its attendant discomforts.

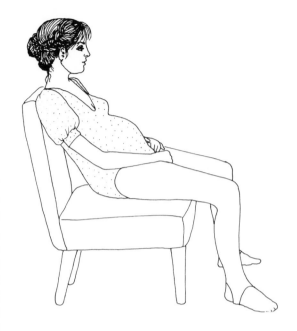

Fig. 1   A *poor sitting posture.*

Whenever you sit at a desk, business machine, sewing machine or table, try not to slouch or indulge in faulty posture of any kind. Instead, try to be aware of how you are holding your body. Sit conveniently near your working area which should be of comfortable height. If possible, have your feet resting on a box or stool, and hold yourself naturally erect.

Sitting on a cushion

1. Place a fairly plump cushion (perhaps one from a chesterfield) on the floor near a wall. Sit down on it and bring your legs toward your body. Keep the legs sufficiently separated to accommodate the abdomen, and position the soles of the feet flat on the floor. Keep the toes relaxed.

2. Lean slightly forward and either hug the knees or rest the arms on them, whichever is more convenient (Fig. 3). For some of you this position could prove quite

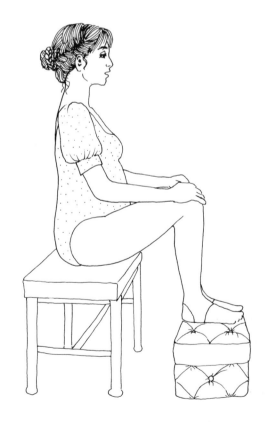

Fig. 2   A *good sitting position. Resting the feet on a prop helps relax the back.*

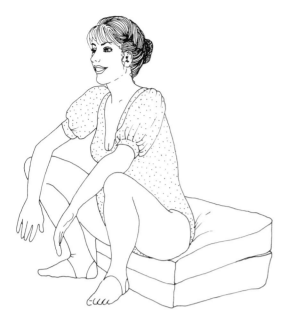

Fig. 3 Sitting on a fat cushion, legs bent and widely separated, can be very comfortable.

comfortable and relaxing to the back. Here again the arch in the lower back is considerably reduced.

Lying Down

The following is a suggested lying position which gives maximum physical relaxation:

1. Lie on your side with your head on one or more pillows. Tuck in your chin and draw your knees toward it. You must be absolutely comfortable, so draw the legs only as far as you can without the slightest strain. What you are in fact achieving in this position is 'straightening out' the curves of the spine and thus relaxing the whole back. If possible and comfortable, it is suggested that you try to have the lower knee closer to the chin than the one above (Fig. 4). This position will help prevent you from rolling onto your face because it gives stability. You will also experience better alignment of the body. Pillows may be placed wherever two bony prominences touch each other, such as the ankles and knees. Pressure from the upper limb or joint on the lower part of the body will thus be alleviated.

2. Fold your arms to make a 'pillow' on which to rest your head (Fig. 4), or arrange them as you find most comfortable. Do not hesitate to make little adjustments here and there to achieve maximum comfort, providing you keep good body alignment.

Notes

Yoga favours lying on the right side. Less pressure appears to be placed on the heart

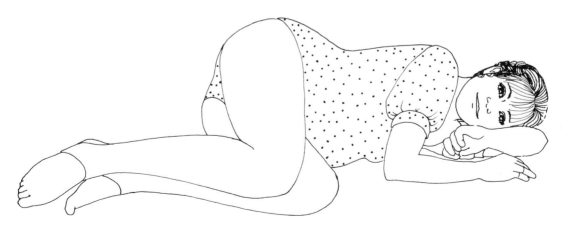

Fig. 4 A comfortable lying position with the lower knee closer to the chest, the back relaxed.

which, in pregnancy, is carrying an extra burden. Of course, you should not lie in the same position indefinitely, so experiment with different body positions.

Whenever you use pillows under or between the limbs, please make quite sure that there is no pressure directly behind the knees or on the calf muscles. This could lead to circulatory problems.

Alternate lying position

Towards the end of pregnancy it is best not to lie on the back for any length of time. The uterus has become quite heavy and its weight on large blood vessels can interfere with the blood circulation and produce certain undesirable conditions. One of these is a lowered blood pressure and a consequent feeling of faintness on suddenly coming to a sitting or standing position. Another side effect of pressure by the heavy uterus on the blood vessels is swelling of the feet due to a slowing down of the return blood flow to the heart and kidneys.

Shortness of breath when lying on the back is another distressing symptom occurring late in pregnancy. The problem occurs because the enlarged uterus presses upward on the diaphragm which in turn encroaches upon the lungs, reducing their capacity for proper expansion. Difficulty in breathing follows.

To reduce the incidence of these conditions, I suggest you use a semi-recumbent (half lying, half sitting) position, with several pillows or cushions behind you for support and comfort. The pillows may also be arranged like an arm-chair so that you can rest your arms more comfortably.

Getting up

When pregnant, getting up from a lying position can be quite an awkward manoeuvre. Here's a way that requires a minimum of effort and strain on the back:

1. Gently slide your body as near to the edge of the bed as is safe.

2. Roll gently onto your side and adopt a position similar to that depicted in Fig. 4.

3. Place the arms in front of the body and use them to push yourself up, very slowly and carefully, until you are resting on one hip (Fig. 5). By using your arms and hands to help you up, you are relieving your back of possible strain.

4. When you are as upright as the length of your arms will permit, place the upper hand on the bed (or floor, depending on where you are lying) beside the upper hip and, still using the arms and hands to assist you, slowly pivot yourself until you are sitting on the edge of the bed with the legs dangling over it.

5. Sit quietly for a minute or so, breathing comfortably, and composing yourself before attempting to stand up. You will give your body a chance to adjust itself, by degrees, to a change of position. Sometimes if you get up too quickly from a lying position, you may feel faint because of a rapid change of blood pressure.

6. To stand up, gently incline your body forward, pressing against the bed with your hands and feeling the floor firmly beneath your feet. Use your hands and the large muscles of your legs to assist you in finally coming to a standing position. Tuck your bottom in, tilting the pelvis slightly forward, and observe correct posture.

Standing

As far as possible, you should try to stand only when you need to go from one place to another. Standing as we usually do, does not in itself promote relaxation, so a good rule to follow is never stand when you can sit, and try to lie instead of sit whenever practicable,

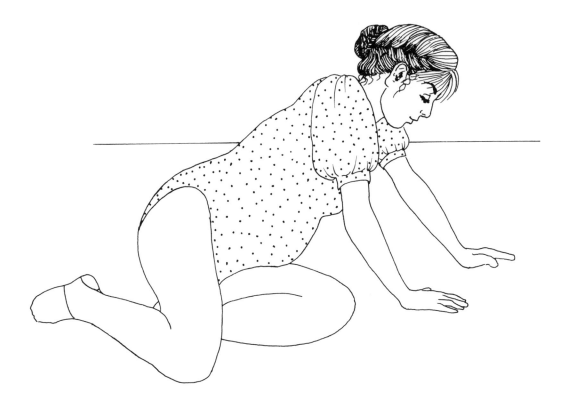

Fig. 5 *Getting up from a lying position need neither be awkward nor strenuous.*

unless you intend to use one of the cross-legged positions or squat.

When you stand, the curves of the spine tend to be accentuated, especially if posture is not good. The part of the intervertebral discs which lies on the inside of these curves receives greater pressure than the part lying near the outside. Continued pressure over a long period of time results in wear and tear of the discs, and eventual pressure on nerves which branch off the spinal column. The greater the curvature of the spine, the greater the pressure on the discs within the curve, and the greater the strain on the muscles and ligaments which support the spine. Therefore, by training yourself to adopt positions whereby these spinal curves are reduced, you would be relieving the intervertebral discs of pressure, and the muscles and ligaments of the back of unwarranted strain.

Whenever you find it necessary to stand,

place one foot flat on a chair, stool, box or other suitable prop, so that the bent knee is on a plane which is considerably higher than that of the hips (Fig. 6). Use this stance when answering the telephone, providing you will not be talking for a long time, in which case you would do better to sit. When ironing you can follow the same procedure. If you must stand, then rest one foot on a box or stool, but it would be preferable to sit, especially if you have much ironing to do.

Many tasks which are done while standing could be done with greater conservation of energy if they were to be done while sitting. Invest in a kitchen stool of suitable height, and use it as much as possible. If you can place your feet on something as well, so much the better. You will be amazed at how much less tired you feel even though you may be working longer and accomplishing more.

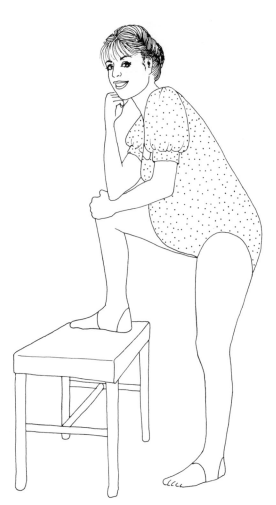

Fig. 6   *Put one foot on a prop when you must stand. It helps reduce back strain.*

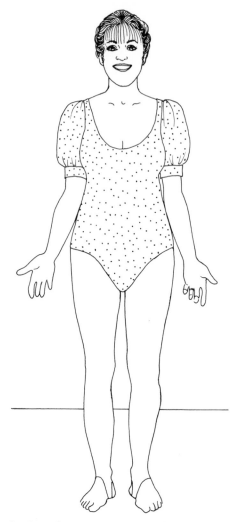

Fig. 7   *A good stance in preparation for walking. Elbows are to the back.*

Walking

Walking is one of the best forms of outdoor exercise in which a pregnant woman can engage. Whenever possible, you should walk every day. Try always to be aware of your carriage as you walk and hold yourself correctly. You will be keeping fatigue to a minimum. Practise the Walking Breath for part of your walk (section 8).

Here is a way of standing which will perhaps give you some idea of how to hold your body correctly in preparation for walking. Stand tall with the palms of the hands 'facing' forward (Fig. 7). In doing this the upper part of the forearms also turn forward, the elbows turn backward and rest near the body, and if you are standing naturally erect your shoulderblades will flatten, and any roundness of the shoulders will be eliminated. Tuck in your bottom so as to tilt your pelvis slightly forward and reduce the arch in the lower back (Fig. 8). If you feel self-conscious about walking this way, rotate the wrists so that the palms are toward the body, but do not change the position of the upper arms.

Try walking this way around the house and

up and down the stairs. In my country of origin I often saw women walking in this manner on their way to market, usually with a basket of fruit or other merchandise upon their head. Sometimes one arm would be raised, and the hand would be resting against the basket if there was any tendency for it to topple; but often no hand would be used. The arm or arms alongside the body would invariably 'face' forward. Even in those days I recall my admiration for the excellent carriage of these market women.

When walking upstairs, try placing the entire sole of the foot on the stair, instead of taking the weight on part of the foot only. You may find that this is less tiring and less likely to leave you short of breath.

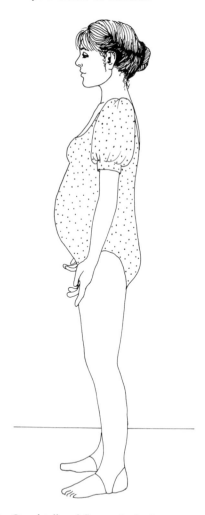

Fig. 8   Stand tall and flatten the back.

Carrying parcels

Avoid carrying anything heavy. If you need to carry heavy objects, divide them so that the total weight is equally distributed between the hands, and let your arms do some work toward sparing the back of possible strain. Do not hunch the shoulders. Hold yourself comfortably erect and be aware of your posture.

Bending down

Use the large muscles of the legs to take your weight and bend at the knees while lowering your body toward an object. Keep your back straight but not rigid. One excellent method of bending to pick up a fallen object or attend to a small child is to bring yourself to a squatting position (Fig. 18, p.87). Stand with the legs well apart then slowly come down, inclining slightly forward, until the buttocks rest near or on the heels. Use your arms and hands for balance and/or support. Hold on to a stable piece of furniture with one hand if that helps.

Whatever method you use when bending down, never bend forward from the waist and allow the back to take the strain. Bend instead at the knees, keeping the back well aligned, and taking most of the weight on your legs. Use your breath to support your movements. The habit of combining breathing with movement will help you conserve energy.

Lifting

It is not a good idea to bend forward from the waist, relying heavily on the muscles of the back, when about to lift something. Lower yourself as if to squat, bring the object you want to lift (for example, a basket of laundry) to about chest level, then, depending greatly on the powerful muscles of the legs, stand up slowly maintaining your hold on the object at chest level. Keep your back straight and use your breath to help you — inhale as you get up.

Reaching

While it is not harmful to stretch upward to one's comfortable limit, it is not recommended that you overreach. It would be too much strain on your back. When you want to get something which is beyond your comfortable reach, use a stool, box or chair on which to climb. The object on which you stand must be stable and strong enough to take your weight. Hold on to something with one hand if necessary. Inhale as deeply as possible as you reach upward.

Chapter 5

The Pelvis and Pelvic Care

The bony pelvis

The pelvis is situated at the lower end of the vertebral column. It is formed by two innominate (hip) bones at the sides, the sacrum (five fused vertebrae) at the back, and the coccyx ('tailbone') which is usually made up of four fused bones. The coccyx is located directly beneath the sacrum. Joints are formed where the hip bones meet the sacrum at the back (sacroiliac joints), where the sacrum meets the coccyx (sacro-coccygeal joint), and where branches of the innominate bones meet in front (symphysis pubis). There are also ligaments or bands of fibrous tissue connecting the bones which form joints.

The functions of the bony pelvis are essentially to house and give production to the pelvic organs (these include the uterus and its attachments, the bladder, and the lower part of the large intestine known as the rectum), and to transmit the weight of the body to the legs.

The pelvic floor

The pelvic floor is situated at the bottom of the pelvis and forms a sling-like support for the pelvic organs. Part of this floor (the perineum) may be seen externally as that area between the thighs and between the anus and the vagina. There are three openings in the pelvic floor, namely, the anus which is the opening of the end of the large intestine or bowel, the vagina leading from the neck of the uterus, and the urethra leading from the bladder for the passage of urine. Each of these orifices is opened and closed by a sphincter (ring-like) muscle, but each sphincter is part of a single large muscle which is made up of fibres arranged in a double figure-eight manner. This muscle is called the *levator ani* and is the main support of the pelvic organs.

During childbirth the pelvic floor muscles are stretched enormously, so much so that the perineal body (the perineum forms the base of the perineal body) which is normally a thick, wedge-shaped mass, becomes very thin tissue. With each successive birth there tends to be a corresponding loss of tone in these muscles, due to extensive stretching. One major function of the pelvic floor is to keep the pelvic organs in their correct position — indeed it is the chief support of the uterus. The gross stretching of the pelvic floor muscles during repeated childbearing can cause these muscles to weaken and become inefficient supports for the uterus and other pelvic organs. Unless these supporting muscles are kept healthy and elastic, uterine prolapse (falling downward of the uterus) and related signs and symptoms can result.

Another function of the pelvic floor is to help the body resist changes in pressure within the abdominal and pelvic cavities during activities which cause an increase of pressure, such as laughing, coughing, sneezing, etc. If the pelvic floor muscles are not kept in good tone but allowed to weaken and become lax, a very disturbing condition can and frequently does result. In gynaecological circles it is called 'stress incontinence of urine', and means that urine trickles away whenever the woman coughs, sneezes, laughs, etc.

Understandably, it is of the utmost importance to endeavour to develop and maintain a healthy pelvic floor in which the muscles are strong, elastic, and of good tone. This is especially desirable in pregnancy where the enlarging uterus places greater strain on its supporting pelvic floor. Apart from maintaining good muscle tone, a woman should learn how to relax her pelvic floor. A rigid perineum can result in a tear or laceration as the baby's head is being born. A laceration is not as easy to repair as a straight incision (episiotomy) which is sometimes made by the doctor to facilitate the passage of the baby's head through the outlet of the birth canal. Actually, when you think about it, 'pelvic floor' is not a very suitable description for an area which we want to keep elastic, and to be able to relax and control at appropriate times. It suggests something rigid, which is the opposite of what is desired. It is, however, an accepted term long in use.

The postures and techniques for this section have been selected for their effectiveness in stretching and toning the muscles of the pelvic floor, helping to make them more efficient as a support for the pelvic organs during pregnancy and following childbirth. They help to improve the blood circulation to this area, keeping at a minimum congestion caused by the increasing weight of the uterus on pelvic blood vessels. They will help to relieve conditions which can arise from such congestion, for example haemorrhoids (piles). They therefore contribute in no small way to a more comfortable pregnancy. Some of the techniques will also help toward acquiring a more elastic pelvic floor, controlling, and relaxing it when necessary. If you can control your pelvic floor muscles satisfactorily as the baby's head is being born, they will offer less resistance to the head, and birth will be smoother. There will

also be less likelihood of your perineum being torn. Finally, these techniques, practised faithfully, will help reduce discomforts which might otherwise occur immediately following childbirth.

Before proceeding to describe the exercises, here is something interesting to ponder. It has been observed that as the muscles of the face tighten, so do those of the pelvic floor. There appears to be a definite relationship between these sets of muscles, even though they are so remotely situated from each other. The chances are that if your facial muscles relax, so will those of your pelvic floor. Therefore, whenever you do movements which involve the pelvic floor muscles, indeed when doing any of the asanas (with the exception of the Lion), try to be aware of what your facial muscles are doing. If you find that, because you are keenly concentrating on a particular movement or holding a position, your face is beginning to tighten, your lips to be compressed, your lower jaw to clench, or your forehead to wrinkle, immediately begin to smooth away these undesirable facial expressions, and compose your features instead. Smile if you feel like it. Let the awareness of facial relaxation be with you as you perform your postures. Developing the habit of facial relaxation will be invaluable to you in labour and indeed throughout life.

Controlling the muscles of the pelvic floor

Earlier in this chapter it was stated that the pelvic floor was perforated in three places by the anus, the vagina, and the urethra, and that these openings were closed and opened by sphincter muscles under the control of the levator ani muscle. However, although these sphincters are part of this larger muscle, it is possible to control each of them independently of the others, or at least with little movement from them.

It has been proved that if the muscles of the

pelvic floor (of which the above mentioned structures are part) are regularly exercised to preserve their tone, stress incontinence of urine, haemorrhoids, itching and/or soreness of the vaginal lining, to name only a few distressing conditions, are much less likely to occur. If you are having your first baby, they may even be avoided altogether.

The exercise which follows is invaluable, not only during pregnancy, but after childbirth, and indeed at all other times, and should be practised more than once daily by all women. Since no one can see you doing it, you can practise it even in public — while waiting for the bus, standing in line at the grocery store, while washing dishes or watching television. One eminent obstetrician/gynaecologist for whom I once worked never failed to instruct his patients in this technique whenever they came back to see him about six weeks after the birth of their baby. He had two main reasons for this. During childbirth the muscles of the pelvic floor undergo immense stretching, and so lose much of their previous tone. Thus, they cannot support adequately the pelvic organs. Consequently, a slight falling downward (prolapse) of these organs may result until the supporting muscles are strengthened through exercise, and regain as much of their former tone as possible. If such exercise is not carried out, various distressing conditions, some of which have already been mentioned, may occur. Not a few women who have borne several children without keeping their pelvic floor muscles in tone have had to have their uterus removed because of the extent of the prolapse. Practise Aswini Mudra (p.106) and be confident that the stretched muscles will quickly regain good tone — indeed tone may even be improved.

The second reason for regular practice of this technique is that many partners claim that sexual intercourse is less pleasurable to them after women have had a baby, because the vaginal muscles feel very slack. Some women, too, note a decrease in the satisfaction they once gained during intercourse for this very reason. The alternate contracting and releasing of the sphincter muscles in Aswini Mudra will firm and tone the muscles of the entire pelvic floor, and reduce the chances of such an occurrence in your relationship with your mate.

As part of your prenatal programme, practise this technique to help you gain control of your pelvic floor, so that during the expulsive stage of labour (when the baby's head is literally being pushed out of the birth canal) you will be able to contribute positively to minimizing the resistance offered by the muscles of your pelvic floor to your baby's head. This will make for a smoother, less prolonged birth, with less likelihood of your perineum tearing.

Immediately following childbirth, Aswini Mudra, done regularly, will improve the blood circulation to your perineum, thus reducing the chances of fluid collecting between the stitches of your episiotomy (an epsiotomy is sometimes unavoidable), and delaying the healing process. It will help keep your perineum supple, and keep to a minimum or prevent altogether any difficulties which may arise when you pass urine or have a bowel movement.

Last, but by no means least, it will help firm the muscles stretched during childbirth. A firm pelvic floor gives a woman a feeling of self-confidence and poise.

Chapter 6

Tension and Relaxation

Tension comes in many forms and from many sources, some of which may not be obvious. In fact, tension can originate in areas of the body which may seem unrelated to that part of it where it is finally most felt. For example, a tired or aching back may be due to weak or tired feet. Consider that the feet bear the entire weight of the body. If they are not strong, or if they do not share equally in bearing this weight, the back muscles will take some of the strain and tighten in an effort to compensate. As tension builds up, the back will become increasingly tired and may even hurt. Think also about tired eyes or eyestrain. Have you ever reflected that these conditions can result in both physical and mental fatigue? Some authorities state that as much as 60 per cent of our mental energy is utilized through our sight. Small wonder then that tired eyes do contribute to much of our tension and fatigue.

Pregnant women must never allow themselves to become over-tired. They should try to anticipate fatigue and take measures to forestall it. Pregnant women do tire easily, and so it is very important that they have frequent rest periods throughout the day and create opportunities for relaxation. As pregnancy advances, the pregnant woman will find that these periods of relaxation will need to be longer and more frequent.

Apart from actual rest periods, there are several measures that can be taken to reduce tension and decrease the stress of fatigue. Try to sit whenever possible while doing certain household tasks. Be sure that work areas are at a height that will ensure comfort and not put strain on your back or shoulders. There are many things that can be done while sitting cross-legged on the floor or squatting (see chapter 2). In such positions you have the added benefits which come from stretching the pelvic floor muscles and holding the spine naturally erect.

Sit or lie with the legs elevated as many times daily as you can. The blood circulation to the legs is benefited, and the whole body made to feel more rested.

Try to cultivate habits of good posture and body movement in all your activities. (Refer to chapter 4 for more detailed information.) Sit, stand and walk tall to reduce harmful stress; never stand when you can squat or sit, and lie down whenever possible.

When concentrating on doing something, are your shoulders hunched and your forehead wrinkled? Try always to keep your body erect but relaxed, and your facial muscles composed. The habit of facial relaxation is well worth cultivating as it has a bearing on the relaxation of the pelvic floor muscles (refer to chapter 5). The relaxation of muscles not directly involved in a particular activity enables you to utilize your energy more efficiently.

Finally, try to develop what is known as economy of movement (and therefore economy of energy). For example, when preparing to bake bread or a cake, do you first assemble all your equipment and ingredients so that they are conveniently near, or do you have to make repeated trips to cupboards for things you have forgotten? These extra trips can easily be avoided if you first plan carefully what you need for the job. This will be a help toward reducing fatigue.

In the section corresponding to this chapter (pp.109-117) techniques are described to help you learn how to conserve that vital energy needed throughout your pregnancy, and especially during labour if you intend to take a truly active part in helping bring your baby into the world. These techniques will help you learn the art of relaxing totally — and it is indeed an art, or, more accurately still, a neuromuscular skill because the muscles are under the control of the nervous system.

Eye exercises

Earlier in this chapter I mentioned that the eyes can utilize up to 60 per cent of your mental energy. You can, therefore, sometimes reduce total body tension enormously by relaxing the eyes. Always have adequate lighting to your work area, and whenever doing close work such as sewing, writing or reading for any length of time, take periodic breaks to rest the eyes. At such times look at a distant object to provide a change of focus. Whenever you go into the country or up the hills or mountains, look far away. We seem to use our eyes mostly for close work, but seldom for looking at a distance.

To strengthen the muscles of the eyes and to relax them, practise circling them, as described in step 14, technique 1 of the Sponge (p.111). Follow this with Palming (p.113).

The feet

Tired feet can make the whole body feel weary. The feet bear the entire weight of the body and should, ideally, share equally in distributing this weight. The extra weight gained in pregnancy puts a greater burden on the feet, and it is even more important at this time that correct posture habits be applied when standing and walking. Take care of your feet and they will serve you well. Do not wait until they ache before giving them due attention.

Exercise the small muscles of the feet by walking barefoot whenever possible, provided that you are walking on a surface which is pliant, such as grass, carpet, or the beach. Walking on hard, rigid surfaces such as hardwood floors and sidewalks is conducive to fatigue and should be avoided.

Walking is excellent at any time, but especially when pregnant and just after childbirth. Pay attention to your posture (refer to chapter 4), and practise the Walking Breath (see section 8) for part of the walk. When walking upstairs, try using the entire soles of the feet rather than walking only on tiptoe. This will help to keep back strain to a minimum, and you will find that you are less short of breath when you reach the top of the stairs. Elevate your legs on a piece of furniture whenever you sit, so as to rest them and afford the valves in the blood vessels a welcome respite. Be careful, however, not to have any pressure on the calf muscles or the areas behind the knees, as that would impede the blood circulation.

One last point of importance — choose your maternity shoes as carefully as you choose your other clothing. Buy shoes in which the heels are neither high nor flat, but comfortably low. Do your shopping for these toward the end of the day when a certain amount of swelling of the feet is not uncommon. If you are fitted in the morning, the shoes may be too tight by the afternoon or evening.

Exercises for the feet

The sitting postures (section 2) are excellent for strengthening the ankles, feet and legs. Remember, however, that those of you with varicose veins should not use most of them. Only the Sitting Warrior and the dynamic variation of the Squatting Pose are permissible.

The hands

Many people find it difficult to rest their hands quietly — even when simply sitting. Some people fidget with their fingers, others must hold a cigarette, still others clutch at the furniture on which they sit or lie. The next time you answer the telephone, observe whether you hold the receiver in a secure but relaxed way or clutch it instead. If you clutch it, you are wasting energy.

When driving your car, hold the steering wheel in a firm but relaxed manner rather than gripping it tensely. The accumulation of tension in the fingers and hands is insidious and difficult to eliminate, so develop the habit of relaxing them whenever they are not doing something constructive.

The Bust Exercise (Fig. 50, p.123) is helpful in getting rid of tension from the fingers and hands. Here are some other movements with similar benefits:

1. Shake the hands loosely as if to rid them of drops of water. Observe the tingling sensation which follows.

2. Using the thumb of one hand, bend each finger of the other toward the palm, then release it. Relax. Repeat with the other hand.

3. Making a 'V' of the index and middle fingers of one hand, place it against each finger of the other and gently push it toward the back of the hand. Release. Relax. Repeat with the other hand.

Sleep

Ideally, sleep should be a state in which the body obtains rest and refreshment after the activities of the day. If sleep has been restful, one awakes feeling revitalized. However, this is not always the case, and it is not uncommon during pregnancy to find that sleep is fitful and of poor quality. If you are experiencing some insomnia, it may be well for you to consider the following, applying them where necessary. Remember that it is not the number of hours of sleep that are significant, but the quality of that sleep.

Position of the bed

The body is regarded as a magnetic field. It should, therefore, lie in a position that is in harmony with the magnetic current of the earth. It is suggested that, especially if you are a very sensitive person, you sleep with your head to the north and your feet to the south. If the idea seems ridiculous but all else fails to remedy insomnia, try this. You may be delightfully surprised!

Food and drink

Avoid eating a heavy meal close to bedtime. The body may be too tired to digest such a meal adequately. Indigestion and consequently disturbed sleep may result. The same caution applies to stimulating drinks such as tea, coffee and even cocoa (herb teas are the exception), providing you have proven that these beverages do keep you from sleeping.

Heating and ventilation

The room where you sleep should be well aired but not draughty. It should be comfortably cool or warm, as best tolerated.

Firmness of your sleeping surface

Firmness of the sleeping surface is important. It should not be rigid. Your back must be given good support, yet the surface on which you lie should be sufficiently pliant.

Your clothing

Your sleeping garments should be kept to a minimum, but loose-fitting and adequately cool or warm, depending on the weather.

Sleeping in the nude, if it suits you, is not a bad idea. It allows the body a chance to breathe, free from the restrictions of clothing to which it is subjected for so many hours of the day.

Bedclothing

This should be light and sufficiently warm. Too many and too heavy blankets place unhealthy pressure on the legs, abdomen and chest. Blood circulation and proper breathing are hindered.

Time to go to bed

The body usually dictates when it's time to sleep; do not protest. Our body is often wiser than we give it credit for. Some people believe that sleep before midnight is more refreshing than that begun after. Remember that each of us is a unique individual.

Position of the body

The position chosen should be very comfortable while keeping the spine in good alignment, to reduce chances of lower back strain. Some people prefer to lie mostly on the left side, while others feel more secure on the right. Yoga favours the right lateral position because it supposedly subjects the heart to less pressure and also opens the left nostril to permit a free flow of spiritual energies. Do not hesitate to place pillows between the knees, ankles, or anywhere else you may wish for added comfort. No pressure should be exerted on the calf muscles or behind the knees. Later in pregnancy you may be more comfortable in an almost upright position which affords easier breathing. Experiment to find the best positions.

Excitement before bedtime

Television programmes of a disturbing nature, or literature that is too stimulating may make you overexcited. Beware of these if you have found that they affect the quality of your sleep adversely.

Breathing and relaxation

Deep, slow, rhythmical breathing, especially in front of an open window if the weather permits, can help induce sound sleep. The Alternate Nostril Breath is very soothing, and the Sponge is excellent for putting you in a suitable state for enjoying sleep at its most refreshing.

State of mind

Try to put the cares of the day from your mind as you prepare for bed. Let go of anxiety or thoughts of fear and hatred. Clear up misunderstandings, and forgive wrong doings, imagined or real, born of short-comings such as we ourselves possess. How can peaceful sleep be obtained if the mind is troubled? Still the mind first.

Waking up

Never get out of bed suddenly. Give the body ample opportunity to accommodate itself to a change of position, and gently prepare it for the day's activities. It has been relatively inactive for many hours. Here is a suggested waking up routine:

Stretch your whole body slowly and leisurely while still in bed. Push the heels away from you, bringing the toes toward you. Stretch the arms upward or sideways. Hold. Release. Bend the knees, placing the soles of the feet on the bed, and press the small of the back firmly against it as you exhale. Hold this position as long as your exhalation lasts. Inhale and relax the muscles. Alternating the legs, circle the ankle clockwise a few times then counterclockwise the same number of times. Relax. Turn onto your side and slowly get up (refer to Fig. 5, p.27). Sit for several seconds to allow your body to adjust to a change from a horizontal to an upright position. By doing this, you will risk less chance of dizziness. Take a few slow, comfortable breaths. Stand up slowly. Do the Standing Pose (Fig. 34, p.101). Relax. Now. proceed with your usual morning routine. If this is the time of day you practise your yoga postures, prepare to do them following your morning toilet. Have a healthy, happy day!

Chapter 7

The Breasts

The increased size and weight of the breasts during pregnancy place greater strain on their underlying supporting muscles. Should these muscles not be kept in good tone through suitable, regular exercise, they will lose their elasticity and ability to support the bust. Following childbirth and lactation, a sagging bustline will result, and this is one thing which causes a woman to look and feel much older than she actually is. Do wear a well-designed, well-fitting brassiere to help support the enlarging breasts, both during pregnancy and during the time when you will be nursing your baby (a nursing brassiere is useful). However, a brassiere, no matter how well made, is not substitute enough for firm underlying muscles. Full dependency on a brassiere can, in fact, contribute to weakening the muscles. It would be much wiser to work at toning, strengthening, and firming the muscular supports of the breasts.

The following muscles support the breasts: 1) The pectoral muscles (pectoralis major and minor) which run across the front of the chest and insert into the bone of the upper arm — whenever you move the arms sideways or bring them across the front of the chest, these muscles are brought into play. 2) Running mainly over the sides of the chest and inserting into the shoulderblades are a group of muscles (serratus magnus) which are exercised during movements of pushing. 3) Finally, there are the intercostal muscles located between the ribs. They are thought to act as elastic supports during respiration.

The selection of postures offered for this chapter (pp.119-123) will exercise these muscle groups. Although you need not practise them all during any one exercise session, you should do one or two of them daily, varying your selection so that, say over a weekly period, you will have covered all of them, after which you return to the one or ones you practised first, and so on.

At this point I should like to remind you that, in addition to practising specific exercises to maintain a firm and healthy bust, you should continue at all times to be aware of the way in which you are holding yourself and performing all your movements, no matter what the activity in which you are involved. Good posture and carriage are essential to a good bustline — no stooping shoulders, no bottom sticking out! Hold yourself naturally erect, keep the shoulder-blades back, and tuck the bottom in.

The function of the breasts is essentially to secrete suitable nourishment (lactation) for the baby during its early life after birth. The decision whether or not to breast-feed your baby should ultimately be yours, and no pressure should be brought to bear upon you in making a decision in so important and intimate a matter. However, do ponder over the fact that breast-feeding does appear to contribute to a more rapid involution (diminution in size of the uterus). As the baby nurses, uterine contractions are stimulated and help bring about this rapid decrease in size.

Here are some limbering-up movements to do before practising the asanas. Sit comfortably, cross-legged or otherwise, remembering to keep the body erect. Relax the arms, hands and shoulders. Establish a comfortable breathing pattern. Now rotate both shoulders backward, squeezing the shoulderblades together, then bring them forward. Keep the facial muscles relaxed. Perform these rotary movements about three times, then change direction, rotating in a forward to backward manner the same number of times. Relax. You are now ready for the asanas.

Chapter 8

The Respiratory System and Breathing

It is by means of the respiratory system that every cell of the body receives its supply of oxygen, and at the same time gets rid of the waste products of oxidation. The oxygen breathed in combines with the carbon and hydrogen of the tissues, enabling the metabolic process of each individual cell to proceed. The waste products of metabolism are eliminated in the form of carbon dioxide and water. Respiration is a two-fold process:

1. Internal or tissue respiration, where there is an interchange of gasses in the tissues.

2. External or pulmonary respiration, where this interchange occurs in the lungs. It is with this part of respiration, of which we can be aware, that we shall deal.

Structures involved in respiration

As we inhale, hopefully through the nostrils, the air passes through the nasal passages into the pharynx (at the back of the mouth), larynx (voice-box), trachea (wind-pipe), left and right bronchi (branches of the wind-pipe), and into the left and right lungs. The bronchi themselves divide into smaller tubes (bronchioles) which terminate in millions of alveoli (air sacs) fed by a network of minute blood vessels.

The lungs themselves are composed of spongy tissue and are covered by a double layer of membrane (pleura). There are two lungs, one on each side of the heart to which they are connected by blood vessels, and with which they work very closely. Other parts of the respiratory system are the neck, thorax (chest cavity), and the abdominal muscles which include the diaphragm.

The thorax is formed by the sternum (breast-bone) which lies between the breasts, part of the spinal column at the back, the ribs and intercostal (between the ribs) muscles at the sides, the diaphragm at the bottom, and the neck at the top.

The diaphragm is a strong, dome-shaped muscle which forms the floor of the thorax, separating it from the abdominal cavity of which it forms a convex roof. It is attached at the back to the lower vertebrae, in front to the breast-bone, and at the sides to the lower six pairs of ribs. It is the chief muscle of inspiration, it compresses the abdominal organs during childbirth, and assists in the emptying of the bladder and bowel.

It is interesting to note that the height of the diaphragm is greatest when one is lying and least when standing. This partly explains why, especially in the latter months of pregnancy, shortness of breath which sometimes occurs as the woman is lying flat, can be relieved by adopting a more upright position; in this way the diaphragm is lowered and pressure from the diaphragm on the lungs is eased.

Why breathe through the nose?

The hope was expressed earlier that you were in the habit of breathing through your nose. As the inhaled air enters the nostrils it is filtered of impurities by tiny hairs, warmed by contact with its mucous lining, and moistened by evaporation from this lining which is extensive. In addition, the Yogis believe (and Western scientists are now seriously considering as plausible) that the olfactory (smelling) nerve, filaments of which enter the upper nostrils, is responsible for the absorption of *prana* (life-force). Yogis believe that the air contains not only oxygen, but also this life-giving prana, without which no one could survive for even a few seconds. Assuming this to be true, think of how much benefit we would be denying ourselves if we were to breathe, for the most part, through the mouth!

What happens when we breathe?

As we inhale, the air entering the lungs gives up its oxygen which is then absorbed by the blood vessels of the alveoli. In exchange it receives waste matter (carbon dioxide) which is excreted on exhalation. The absorbed oxygen is utilized by the body, through the blood, for the nourishment of every cell.

The importance of proper breathing

The foetus depends on the woman for satisfactory growth and development. Proper oxygenation contributes greatly to the health and well-being of the woman and consequently to that of the foetus. Most of us use only about one-fifth of our potential lung capacity. While this may seem adequate, it is not nearly enough for optimal health, marks of which are abundant energy and a positive attitude to life. In pregnancy we ought to enjoy excellent health because of the greater demands made on our system, and because another life depends on ours. This is a responsibility that should not be taken lightly, and every effort should be made to upgrade our own health so as to enhance the well-being of the foetus. Proper breathing would contribute to this upgrading of health, because it would increase our supply of life-force. Poor posture habits such as slouching, which compresses the internal organs, do not permit proper expansion of the lungs or satisfactory aeration. Correct posture is perhaps the first step toward improving the quality of our breathing. If we were habitually to breathe in the shallow manner that matches incorrect posture, our intake of oxygen and life-force, although seemingly adequate, would not in fact be satisfactory for optimal health. Elimination of waste products through exhalation would be incomplete, some of this waste matter would remain in the bloodstream, and body cells would be recontaminated. Recontamination can and does manifest itself in a variety of ailments such as sluggishness, headaches, and depression. The causes of these and other disorders are not often suspected as being related to poor breathing habits.

Breath and emotions are closely linked. Good emotional balance is very desirable in pregnancy and childbirth. Observe how shallow and irregular your breathing becomes if you are upset, apprehensive or depressed. At such times (hopefully they will be few) hold yourself in a more upright position, for your shoulders are probably drooping, take a few slow, deep, even breaths, and notice a slight change for the better in your state of mind. Alternatively, when you feel happy and at peace, notice the smoothness, depth and regularity of your breathing, and note also that you are probably holding yourself erect and standing tall. Thus body, mind, emotions, and breath are inseparable.

It appears to be true that women seldom go

short of oxygen during pregnancy and childbirth for the following reasons: There is a larger volume of blood circulating; the circulation through the lungs is slower, permitting more thorough oxygenation; the activity of the diaphragm is increased, and this enhances excretion of the waste products of respiration. However, these processes, although adequate to sustain the life of the woman and that of the foetus, do not at this level appear adequate for ensuring relative freedom from illnesses and discomforts, and for vibrant health.

The breathing exercises selected are offered with a view to encouraging women to strengthen and improve their breathing apparatus, and to establish and maintain better breathing habits which, together, will contribute to better health during and after pregnancy. They are given here to help women prepare themselves for using their breath advantageously during labour. They are not, however, actual breathing patterns used in labour. Such patterns are best learnt at a preparation for childbirth class where personal supervision is available.

Some guidelines for practising the breathing exercises

First, *consult your doctor* and obtain his or her permission to practise the simple breathing techniques which follow.

Always breathe through the nose. There will be exceptions to this rule during labour, when you will be sometimes instructed to blow through the mouth, and to pant at other times. However, as a general rule, develop the habit of nose breathing as opposed to mouth breathing. The reasons for this were given earlier in the chapter.

I have purposely refrained from suggesting that you hold your breath during the postures given in this book. As you have discovered, your body is now having to cope with many added burdens, and indiscriminate retention

of the breath could place a strain on the heart which is already working overtime. Being able to hold the breath for a number of seconds, however, is indeed an asset when you are in the second stage of labour. At this time you are literally helping push the baby out of the birth canal, and you will be instructed to take a deep breath, to hold it, and to release it in a controlled manner as you simultaneously push downward. You may find that you need to be able to retain and release your breath in this manner for as long as sixty seconds, depending on the length of the uterine contraction. I therefore suggest that you learn the technique of breath retention under the personal guidance of a qualified teacher at one of the many preparation for childbirth classes now available, or at a childbirth yoga class if you are lucky enough to find one. For the time being, however, the exercises for this section (pp.125-129), if they are done carefully and regularly, will help increase your lung capacity and strengthen your entire breathing apparatus, so that when the time comes you will find it easy to retain and control your breath as instructed.

Always use a comfortable position in which the spine is erect but not rigid, and the body is relaxed. Try to focus on and be aware of the movement of the abdominal muscles in particular. There should also be no obvious movement of the upper chest if you are breathing correctly. Try not to raise the shoulders; they should be relaxed.

Breathe slowly, deeply, and evenly. This type of breathing is conducive to evenness of temper and peace of mind.

Although certain breathing techniques do help to reduce fatigue, it is not a good idea to begin a period set aside specifically for breathing exercises when you are tired. After such a session, you should relax completely for five to ten minutes in the Sponge (section 6).

Take every opportunity to practise breathing exercises out of doors, especially in places where there seems little likelihood of pollution, such as in some parts of the countryside or in the hills or mountains.

Include deep abdominal breathing several

times in your work day. It will help you develop skill in increasing the length of both your inhalation and exhalation, as well as the distance to which your abdominal wall can be raised. You will find the ability to do this of value in labour. You will also be strengthening your diaphragm. Through regular practice of this kind of breathing you will become adept at it, and will better be able to control your breath when under stress (for example, in labour).

Follow the rules already outlined for practising the asanas (chapter 1).

Chapter 9

Minor Discomforts of Pregnancy

During pregnancy several conditions may arise which, although not in themselves serious as a rule, can nevertheless adversely affect one's feeling of well-being. If any of these disorders occur, there are certain measures that can be taken to relieve or correct them in a natural way.

Nausea and vomiting

Among the many changes taking place in the body at this time are hormonal changes and emotional adjustments. These two factors may contribute to the nausea and vomiting which occurs during the first three or four months of pregnancy. Here are some suggestions for relieving these:

Never allow the stomach to become empty. The lowered level of blood sugar which occurs at such times seems to aggravate a tendency to nausea. Have fresh fruit available for snacking. In addition to providing vitamins, it provides natural sugar which is quickly assimilated and converted into blood sugar. Put a plain, wholewheat cracker on your bedside table, ready to eat, if necessary, first thing in the morning. Since nausea is sometimes related to a deficiency of the vitamin B complex, try to ensure an adequate daily intake of this nutrient (chapter 12 gives some natural sources).

Never get out of bed suddenly. On awaking, lie quietly for several minutes, practising gentle, rhythmic breathing or another relaxation technique. Get up very slowly, and prepare for the day in a leisurely fashion.

Never overeat. Keep meals smaller, plainer and lighter. Chew food slowly and thoroughly. Drink beverages between rather than with meals.

Spearmint or red raspberry leaf tea, sipped slowly, is useful in relieving nausea and vomiting.

Indigestion and heartburn

The top of the stomach through which food enters is opened and closed by a sphincter muscle called the cardiac sphincter. Due to the circulation in the body of certain hormones during pregnancy, there may be times when this muscle is relaxed too much. When this happens, it causes the contents of the stomach along with the stomach acids to bubble back into the oesophagus (gullet), giving rise to a typical burning sensation in the throat and stomach.

To obtain relief from such distressing occurrences, follow the suggestions given in paragraph 2 of the section on nausea and vomiting. Some antacids do appear to give a measure of relief, but you should first consult your doctor before taking any of them. Under no circumstances should you take baking soda in water (see chapter 12 — contra-indications).

Heartburn may also be due to a shortage of B vitamins in the diet, so make sure you are obtaining a sufficient amount daily.

Flatulence

This is usually a result of bacterial action in the intestines, producing excessive gas. Other contributory factors seem to be a reduced quantity of acid in the stomach, and decreased movement of the entire gastro-intestinal tract (referring to stomach and intestines). Here again, hormonal influences seem to be partially responsible. Because of these, gas tends to accumulate, sometimes to an uncomfortable degree. Some relief measures have been suggested in the third paragraph of the section on nausea and vomiting. Others are:

Avoid constipation. Refer to chapter 12 for foods that act as natural laxatives. Do not take commercially prepared laxatives without your doctor's approval.

Although many people prefer to avoid foods such as beans, peas, cabbage, etc., because they believe that these are gas forming, it is not actually true that such foods produce more gas than certain others. It is usually the manner in which these foods are prepared that contributes to gas formation. Cooking them in much water at high temperature causes sulphur compounds to break down. The compounds lead to gas formation during digestion, and it is this which causes discomfort. The problem of gas should not arise if these vegetables are chilled thoroughly, then shredded or diced, heated quickly in the initial stages of cooking, and steamed in very little water at a lower temperature for about eight minutes only.

Unless you have varicose veins, squat as many times daily as you can. Squat, if you can manage this comfortably without losing balance, when you are having a bowel movement, or place a wooden box, low bench, or other suitable aid in front of the toilet so that you can place your feet flat on it. With your feet bracing against such an object and your legs widely separated, you will be able to push more effectively to aid elimination. If you have varicose veins, practise instead the dynamic variation of the Squatting Pose (section 2).

Practise the Knee Press (Wind-relieving Pose) frequently (section 3), and when this condition is particularly troublesome.

Constipation

Hormonal changes also affect peristalsis, the wave-like contraction of the tubular walls of internal organs, which presses their contents onward. The intestines are no exception, and it is partly because their ability to contract is decreased under hormonal influence, that there is a tendency for waste matter to accumulate, leading to constipation. Added to this, the woman may be taking iron supplements which do make some people constipated.

Try the following to gain help in relieving a condition which must definitely be remedied if excellent health is to be maintained:

Refer to and apply the suggestions given in paragraphs four and five of the section on flatulence.

Practise the Complete Breath several times daily, and certainly when out of doors.

Increase your intake of fresh fruit, fresh (raw) vegetables such as celery, green salads, and sprouts such as alfalfa. See chapter 12 for other foods which have a natural laxative action. You are again reminded to avoid taking commercially prepared laxatives unless your doctor has prescribed one.

Make sure your daily vitamin B intake is adequate. A deficiency can contribute to constipation.

Pressure symptoms

In this category fall several conditions which are largely a result of pressure by the enlarging uterus on the pelvic blood vessels. The pressure so produced interferes to some extent with the return flow of blood to the heart and generally slows down the circulation in the blood vessels. Poor posture and lax abdominal muscles worsen the situation. The following five disorders will be considered under this heading:

Swelling of the hands and feet

Body fluids tend to collect in the limbs which hang downward. By elevating the swollen part, fluid is given a chance to redistribute itself (Fig. 45, p.116). Note the absence or reduction of swelling after a night's rest, because the body has been in a horizontal or near horizontal position for several hours.

Sitting too long and too often on a chair, especially with the legs crossed, compresses the large blood vessels to the legs. Swelling can result. Sit, therefore, in one of the sitting positions described in section 2 (p.83), observing any contraindications. Whatever your sitting position, do not remain in any one for too long; a frequent change of position helps maintain good blood circulation. When waiting for the bus, walk back and forth periodically or wiggle the toes. One further word of caution — do not sit with a small child on your legs as this further impedes the circulation.

Adding salt to food seems to contribute to swelling. Salt encourages fluid retention in the body tissues. Some doctors restrict the use of salt in the diet of their pregnant patients. Follow your own doctor's instructions in this matter. Chapter 12 suggests some natural salt substitutes.

Varicose veins

See paragraph 2 in the section on swelling of the hands and feet. Do the Cat Pose (Figs. 19 and 20 only, p.89-90) to give the body temporary relief from an upright position in which the forces of gravity are actually working against an improvement of this condition.

Sit rather than stand while working, resting the feet on a suitable prop. Do the dynamic form of the Squatting Pose (section 2, p.88). The movement of the muscles close to the affected veins helps the blood circulation in those veins to improve. For this very reason

walking is excellent, and you should take a daily walk out of doors, weather permitting.

Never wear restrictive garments around the calves, thighs or waist (such as knee-high socks, garters or belts). They tend to impede blood circulation and aggravate the condition.

Relax for short periods daily with the legs elevated on a piece of furniture or against a wall (Fig. 45).

Read chapter 4. Poor posture, especially one in which the shoulders are hunched and the arch in the small of the back is accentuated, makes varicose veins worse. Remember also that high heels throw the body out of alignment and promote bad posture. Wear shoes with comfortably low heels.

Haemorrhoids (piles)

Haemorrhoids are a form of varicose veins which protrude from the rectum (lower end of the large intestine). They can be very painful, may itch, and even bleed. Any form of medication for their relief should be prescribed by your doctor. Since constipation and consequent straining during bowel movement aggravate the condition, follow the suggestions already given for preventing constipation. Ensure an adequate daily intake of B vitamins; a deficiency may have a bearing on the incidence of haemorrhoids.

The following is a little exercise which gives a beneficial massage to the rectum, but do not attempt it if the haemorrhoids are painful or bleeding: Sit as for the Leg Flop (Fig. 9, p.79). Either hold onto the feet or place the hands on the floor behind you and rock from side to side.

Leg cramps

Pressure from the enlarging uterus on pelvic blood vessels may produce leg cramps. Such cramps may also result from stretching both legs too vigorously, or from a calcium or B vitamin deficiency. Even where the calcium intake is adequate, the phosphorus intake may be proportionately too high, and the excess phosphorus in the blood lowers the amount of calcium with resulting leg cramps. For example, if milk is taken in excessive amounts, the high phosphorus content will outweigh the calcium content, producing a form of muscular spasm which manifests itself as a cramp in the leg. The same is true of nutritional yeast taken excessively (unless the yeast is fortified).

If you suddenly experience such a cramp, bend your ankle by pushing the heel firmly away from you and bringing the toes toward the front of the lower leg. If you are lying down, it sometimes helps if you can manage to stand up. When performing the postures, take care not to overstretch your legs by pointing the toes intensely away from you. When stretching first thing in the morning, the tendency may be to point the toes, but be careful (see suggested waking up routine, chapter 6).

Shortness of breath

This is usually more noticeable toward the end of pregnancy, and is caused by the pressure of the uterus against the diaphragm, which in turn reduces the available space in the chest cavity for the lungs to expand fully. Breathing difficulty may be more evident when lying than when upright, so use as many pillows as necessary to raise the head and shoulders and give them satisfactory support. Raising the arms above the head will promote better expansion of the chest cavity, allowing an improved air intake. The principle of raising the arms above the head to permit better rib cage expansion and consequent easier breathing can be seen in the performance of the Mountain Posture (Fig. 56).

When climbing stairs, do so in an unhurried manner, maintaining good posture and a rhythmical breathing pattern. On reaching the top, rest while trying to re-establish even, comfortable breathing. If you can spare half a minute or so, pause and take a few deep breaths. Raise your arms to shoulder level as you inhale, and lower them as you exhale.

Sometimes shortness of breath, especially if it is coupled with a fatigue that is out of proportion to what you have been doing, can be a sign that you are becoming, or already are, short of iron or B vitamins. In this case, you should tell your doctor about these symptoms. He will have your blood checked, and if necessary, prescribe a remedy that is suitable.

Backache

Here is a common condition which appears to be the curse of so-called civilized nations. Studies have shown, by contrast, that there is little evidence of backache among primitive peoples. In chapter 4 I have considered the problem in some detail, suggesting measures for relief. In chapter 3, body movements are described for use in helping strengthen the muscles of back and abdomen.

Although weak muscles and poor posture contribute greatly to backache, there is yet another cause of it during pregnancy. It is the effect of a hormone called *relaxin* which literally relaxes certain joints and ligaments, for example the sacroiliac joints where the hip bones meet the sacrum at the back. It seems reasonable to suppose, therefore, that strengthening the muscles supporting such joints would help reduce a tendency to backache. It is certainly a more natural approach to dealing with the problem than depending on analgesics (pain-killers) which, in any case, should not be taken without your doctor's knowledge and consent.

Round ligament spasm

The round ligaments are cords composed partly of muscle, partly of connective tissue, and extend from the top corners of the uterus through the groin to insert into the pubic area. As the uterus enlarges and descends farther into the pelvis, it sometimes causes a kinking of these ligaments. When this happens, it produces a spasm which may manifest itself as a 'stitch', usually on the right side, but sometimes on the left.

If such a spasm occurs in public, bend down as if to tie your shoelaces, or bend over and pretend to peer into a shop window. Remain thus, breathing as evenly as possible, until the spasm wears off. It usually does so quickly. If you are indoors, try the Cat Pose (Figs. 19 and 20 only, pp.89-90). You may also try sitting in a cross-legged position (section 2), or lie on your side as depicted in Fig. 4 (p.25).

Motion sickness and dizziness

A sudden change from a lying or near horizontal position to an upright one results in a rapid alteration of the blood pressure and may cause dizziness. Always get up slowly from such a position. This way, the body is given a proper chance to adjust itself to the change, and so does the blood pressure.

Motion sickness can be the result of depleted blood sugar, so do not allow your stomach to become empty. Nibble on fresh fruit which contains natural sugar, readily assimilable and converted into blood sugar. Slow, deep, even breathing when you feel the onset of this symptom can do much to ease it.

Insomnia

Difficulty in sleeping soundly appears to be a common problem of late pregnancy in particular. The causes of insomnia are numerous, and so it is best, in trying to treat this state, to determine the underlying causes first. Please refer to the section on sleep in chapter 6 for possible causes and suggested remedies.

One reason why you may be unable to sleep properly is because the foetus may be particularly active. Try altering your position and see if that helps.

If you are lying awake because of back discomfort or backache, ask your husband to give you a light massage with a pure vegetable oil such as safflower seed oil, and have your pillows rearranged to give better support to your head, shoulders, back and limbs. The massage should prove soothing, relaxing and soporific.

If difficulty in breathing seems to be the cause of sleeplessness, try using a semi-recumbent (half lying, half sitting) position, with pillows supporting head, shoulders and back comfortably. A more upright position will relieve some of the pressure of the diaphragm on the lungs. It will permit better chest and lung expansion. Do the following for half a minute or more: Inhaling slowly, smoothly and as evenly as possible, raise the arms to shoulder level. Exhale in similar fashion as you lower the arms.

Please do not take any sedatives or tranquilizers without your doctor's permission. Chapter 12 suggests some natural tranquilizers which may prove helpful in combating insomnia.

Mood changes

Hormonal changes occurring in pregnancy are thought to be responsible in part for many women's susceptibility to frequent changes of mood. Such changes may cover a wide range from states of elation to states of depression. There are so many adjustments taking place in a woman's body at this time, that it is not surprising if her emotional balance is upset. A woman needs added strength during pregnancy. Yoga, practised faithfully, can do much to contribute to this strength by working on body, mind and emotions, all of which are very closely related. It can help provide the discipline which will be needed to cope with the approaching responsibility of caring for a baby, and making necessary adjustments in the relationship between you and your partner once the baby arrives. If there are already children, it will contribute extra strength for handling added responsibilities. However, by the very nature of her emotional make-up, a woman needs constant reassurance and other forms of emotional support from a loved one. It is here that a husband or other close friend can play a vital role, and should be encouraged to make himself as knowledgeable as possible of the processes of pregnancy and childbirth, so as to be able to give support with insight and understanding. With this help, a woman can enjoy a happy pregnancy, and approach childbirth relaxed and self-confident.

Although there does not always seem to be an apparent reason for a sudden change of mood, it may be worthwhile to look for an underlying cause, especially if such a mood is frequent. For example, if it occurs to you that certain emotional upsets may be related to a deficiency of certain nutrients in your diet, take steps to remedy this. A shortage of the B vitamins can cause depression (this group of vitamins is necessary for sound nerves).

Learn how to obtain them through natural sources (chapter 12 offers a few).

You may need extra iron, more rest, better sleep, or a combination of all. Ask your doctor to check your blood to find out if you need an iron supplement (such as ferrous gluconate or ferrous fumarate), then take only what is prescribed. Certain foods have a rich supply of iron in a natural form, and can be included in the diet (see chapter 12). Refer to chapter 6 for aids to reducing fatigue, relaxing more efficiently, and sleeping better. If you are constantly tired or are not obtaining all the essential nutrients in your daily diet (or both), you are more likely to become irritable and depressed.

Whenever you feel the onset of agitation, irritability, or depression, practise several rounds of the Alternate Nostril Breath (section 8). It will help calm and soothe your nerves. The Rhythmic Breath, described in the same section, is another good standby.

Chapter 10

Caesarean Birth

A caesarean birth is one in which the baby is delivered through incisions in the walls of the abdomen and uterus (caesarean section, or C-section). The word 'caesarean' most likely originates from the Roman law of 715 B.C., *lex caesarea*, which required the performance of abdominal surgery to save the baby of a dead or dying mother.

Reasons for caesareans

There is much speculation as to the precise reasons for the increase in caesarean births. One factor may be the almost universal decision among obstetricians to deliver most first breech babies by this method. Another is that women who were formerly precluded from successful pregnancy — such as those with diabetes or high blood pressure — can now have a chance to bear children. Delivery by caesarean section protects the offspring of such women from trauma that may be encountered in a normal labour.

Caesarean sections are also performed in 35 to 40 per cent of first pregnancies where the woman's pelvic outlet is too small for the baby's head to pass through; when labour is not progressing normally; when the foetus is in distress; in women with heart disease, and in post-mature women, who are two or three weeks past their due date.

Sometimes a caesarean section may be done because the woman has had another child by this method. This does *not* mean, however, that because a woman has had one

caesarean delivery, all subsequent deliveries must be by the same route. It depends why the C-section was necessary in the first instance.

Fallacies

One of the myths about caesarean birth is that 'the typical caesarean woman' is short, small-boned and delicate, with tiny feet. Were this true, then all those diminutive Asian and Oriental women would have their babies by caesarean section.

While I was writing the script for this chapter, I remembered my friend, Bonnie, who had her first baby by caesarean. I first met Bonnie at a yoga class. She's a trained physiotherapist; tall, well-built and very fit looking. After the birth of her child she wrote to me: 'Scott was born October 9 by C-section — elective. He was breech, and I had a narrow pelvic outlet.' (Elective caesarean delivery means that surgery is preplanned and prescheduled because of an existing problem.)

The other glaring fallacy about caesareans is: 'Once a caesarean, always a caesarean.' As mentioned in the previous section of this chapter, one delivery by caesarean section does not necessarily mean that all following deliveries must be by the same route. Some women who have had a caesarean birth have subsequently had a vaginal delivery. Several studies show that 38.5 to 72.5 per cent of women who have had one caesarean birth can safely have a vaginal birth, depending on the reason for the original caesarean.

If you are considering a vaginal birth after having had a caesarean, do *discuss with your doctor* the reasons for your first caesarean, and your wishes for a vaginal delivery this time.

Feelings

It is normal for pregnant women to feel some apprehension about the outcome of their pregnancy. To those facing caesarean delivery, this anxiety can intensify. Among the emotions experienced by women who have had caesarean births are:

● Fear that the baby may be damaged during surgery.

● Fear or re-living a previous painful surgical or related experience.

● Fear of having 'failed' as a woman; of having 'let down the team'.

● Anger for not 'performing' as desired or expected.

● Resentment toward the baby for not 'co-operating', such as in a breech presentation.

Men, too, feel varying degrees of anguish at the prospect of a partner's caesarean birth. They may wonder:

● Will my partner survive?

● Will the baby live?

● Will the baby be normal?

Childbirth educators recommend education and empathy as aids to alleviating these real and powerful emotions. Knowing what to expect and how best to cope are two of the best defences against the stresses of uncertainty and fear.

Do attend a class especially designed for women anticipating caesarean birth, if one is available; otherwise, look for and attend a community-based prenatal class, and encourage your partner to accompany you. Caesarean support groups exist, as well, and if you have access to one, do take advantage of this. In addition, check in your local library or book shop for a good book on caesarean birth. Being informed is one of the best first steps to take forward feeling less uncomfortable and more confident about a forthcoming caesarean delivery.

You're certainly *not* a failure because you're going to have a caesarean section or because you've had one. One-third of all women giving birth will have their babies by the surgical route; it's ridiculous to think of them as failures. Caesarean birth is an alternative method of ushering forth new life.

One woman wrote this to me:

I have had two caesarean sections and the first one was a complete surprise for which I was totally unprepared. Ever since that experience, and in preparation for my second C-section, I have read every article I could find on the subject . . . Every other article had stated that women feel such let-down, failure and helplessness. I had experienced none of those feelings, simply thankfulness for a method of delivering a healthy baby.

Instead of being preoccupied with doubt and self-pity, do try to focus on the positive aspects of the caesarean experience. Your life will be the richer for it.

Before surgery

Apart from emergency operations (suddenly necessitated by medical circumstances, for example), most caesarean births take place, I believe, as a result of careful and concerned medical judgement. Some details of procedure differ from hospital to hospital and from doctor to doctor, but the following are what you can generally expect before surgery.

On the morning of the operation, you may be asked to shower and be given an enema to ensure that your bowel is completely empty. The operative area (usually the lower abdomen) may be shaved and cleansed with an antiseptic solution. A catheter may be introduced into your urinary bladder to keep it empty. The catheterization may be uncomfortable but should not be painful.

You will find the breathing and relaxation exercises you practised prenatally very useful. If you have someone with you, the comfort of his or her presence can reduce apprehension.

Other pre-operative procedures include the taking of your blood pressure, possibly an electrocardiogram (ECG) to check your heart function, and the introduction of a needle, usually into one of your arm veins, to which intravenous apparatus will be attached.

Anaesthesia

Anaesthesia may be either *general*, during which you're 'asleep', that is, unconscious; or it may be *epidural*. In the latter you are awake. The anaesthetic is introduced by injection into the nerve pathways of the lower part of the spine. It produces a temporary loss of sensation below the lower ribs.

To lessen the impact of anaesthesia on your system, do practise breathing and relaxation exercises before surgery. If you have kept your spine flexible in the preceding months by faithfully doing the back exercises and by practising good posture and body mechanics, you should not find it difficult to arch your back ('round' it) for epidural anaesthesia.

Incisions

The incision into the uterus (uterine incision) may be either transverse (also called low segment or horizontal) or classical (vertical). The transverse incision is much more commonly performed now, and is preferred for physiological and safety reasons.

The skin incision may be vertical (midline) or horizontal ('bikini' or Pfannenstiel), and is separate from the uterine incision. The 'bikini' incision goes from side to side, just above the pubic bone. Once the hair grows back, the incision scar is usually hardly visible. This incision is preferred by most women for both comfort and cosmetic reasons. The vertical incision is, however, sometimes used by doctors who feel more comfortable with it, and in certain situations in which it is considered advantageous.

The abdominal incision is closed with catgut, nylon, or silk sutures (stitches); sometimes with metal clips. (These are usually removed between 5 and 7 days after surgery.) The area is covered with a suitable dressing.

Most incisions heal quickly, leaving only a faintly visible line that eventually fades (unless you tend to form raised, or keloid, scars). How your scar ultimately appears will depend on your particular healing ability and the general condition of your skin (hence the importance of proper skin care).

After surgery

After your baby is born, you may spend about three hours in the recovery room where your condition will be closely observed. This is a good time, if circumstances permit it, to establish a bond with your child. If your partner is present, he can ask to hold the baby, too. Here's another excerpt from my friend's letter: 'Tony was out in the hall and had a cuddle before I did and thoroughly revelled in the moment.'

Do try to spend as much time with your baby as you can manage. Don't treat him or her as something fragile. Generally, the only marked difference between a baby born by the caesarean method and one born vaginally is this: the head of the former is usually perfectly formed since there has been no moulding from the pressure of passage through the birth canal.

Breastfeeding

If you plan to breastfeed your baby, do let your doctor know before delivery, if possible. Ask to hold and nurse your infant immediately or soon after the operation (even on the delivery table or in the recovery room), if the doctor agrees and circumstances permit. Remember this: if you wish to breastfeed your baby you can do it, whether you have had a caesarean section or not. Here are some advantages to nursing your child soon after surgery:

● You establish the mother-baby skin contact so vital to successful bonding.

● Your baby receives reassurance by hearing your heartbeat and from the warmth of your body.

● The first breast secretion (colostrum) is rich in nutrients and immunization properties.

● Nursing after a caesarean birth is a natural healer for both body and mind. It helps the uterus return to its non-pregnant size (involute) quickly and satisfactorily. It is one way for some mothers to prove to themselves that, although they did not give birth naturally, they are nevertheless very much a mother and very feminine.

Breastfeeding is no guarantee for protection from pregnancy. At this time, however, don't take an oral contraceptive ('the pill'); wait until baby is weaned. (*See also* the section on sex and contraception later in this chapter, page 58.)

Back on the ward

Most women are up and about the day after they've had a caesarean section. Once back on the ward, you will have your temperature, pulse and blood pressure checked frequently, as well as your vaginal discharge (lochia). Do *report* any heavy or bad-smelling discharge or any large clots. *Don't* use

tampons for at least 4 weeks, and certainly not until your cervix (neck of womb) is completely closed. *Check with your doctor.* Otherwise, you risk infection. Even though you may not have laboured, your cervix will have opened a little.

Aches and pains

The most common problems after caesarean birth are due to lack of mobility and to various physical discomforts. Especially if you're breastfeeding, 'after pains' tend to be more noticeable than otherwise, particularly if this isn't your first baby. Do practise breathing and relaxation exercises faithfully to help you cope effectively with these discomforts.

Gas pains after surgery are not uncommon. They usually abate as you become more mobile. Meanwhile, support your abdomen with both hands and do deep breathing exercises (for example, The Complete Breath in section 8, p.125-126). in addition, try lying on your left side, with your knees bent and pulled toward your chest. Breathe slowly and rhythmically. The Knee Press (Wind-relieving Pose) in section 3, p.91-92, is excellent for ridding the body of troublesome gas. Practise, as well, the abdominal exercises described in the section on Essential Exercises later in this chapter, page 57.

Eating and drinking

Your digestive system is not ready for your usual diet until 24 to 36 hours after surgery. Ask visitors not to bring you food during this time. Surgeons usually prescribe clear fluids to begin with, slowly working up to 'diet as tolerated'.

Once back to your normal diet, do drink plenty of fluids, especially if you're breastfeeding, so as not to become dehydrated. Fluids also help prevent constipation. Be sure to include in your diet lots of vitamin C-rich liquids, such as unsweetened fruit juice. Eat adequately of fresh fruits and vegetables, milk products and whole grain products. They contain nutrients essential for maintaining good health, for promoting healing, and for keeping the skin resilient. Please review chapter 12 (Nutrition Notes).

Essential exercises

As mentioned earlier, in the section entitled 'Back on the ward', most women are up and about the day after a C-section. Early graduated, consistent exercise is important to the healing process and to promote proper union of the incision edges. It is also important to help restore the muscle tone and function of all body structures; to help avoid complications such as pneumonia and blood clots in the legs, and to foster well-being.

Leg and foot exercises

While you're still in bed, even in the recovery room, *ask your doctor or physiotherapist* if you can do the following leg and foot exercises.

1. Wiggle your toes.

2. First point your toes toward the ceiling then toward the bottom of the bed. Do this slowly, several times.

3. Bend one knee and slide the foot up the bed toward you; slide the foot away from you until the leg is again flat on the bed. Do this a few times. Repeat the movements with the other leg.

Later, dangle your legs over the side of the bed and practise rotating the ankles: first clockwise a few times, slowly and with awareness, synchronizing normal breathing with the ankle rotations; then counter-clockwise, in the same manner, the same number of times.

The leg and foot exercises improve circulation in the legs and help prevent thrombophlebitis (inflammation of a vein, usually with the formation of a blood clot).

Abdominal exercises

1. Support your abdomen with your hands. Inhale slowly, smoothly and deeply through your nostrils. Exhale steadily through your mouth, saying 'huff' or 'huh'. (Don't worry; your stitches won't pop.) Do this a few times then repeat the exercise a few more times during the day.

This is a useful breathing exercise if you have had general anaesthesia. It helps rid your system of anaesthetic residues and dislodge mucus that may be present in the lungs. It also helps reduce the amount of gas in your intestines, and improves intestinal motility and abdominal muscle tone.

Whenever you're about to sneeze, laugh, cough, or hiccough, 'splint' your incision by supporting your abdomen with both hands. This will inhibit potentially painful involuntary movement of the abdomen. Remember, too, to continue the good posture and carriage you practised during pregnancy, as best as you can.

Please review chapter 13 and section 9 (post partum), as well as section 6 (tension and relaxation) and section 8 (breathing exercises).

It may be months before your abdominal muscles regain excellent tone. You need to be patient and to persevere with your daily exercises. Don't start exercising enthusi-astically, only to 'forget' to do them after a while, or become 'too busy' for them. Don't be afraid of damaging your incision as this is unlikely to happen. If it hurts as you exercise, go back to the simplest techniques — the breathing exercises for instance — working up gradually to the more challenging ones as you become pain free and stronger.

Exercising does increase the flow of lochia, but if the discharge isn't heavy, don't be unduly concerned.

For best results, be prepared to work conscientiously at regaining figure and function.

Perineal exercises

Some educators believe that it's unnecessary for women who have had a caesarean section to practise pelvic floor exercises. The fact is, however, that although you may not have laboured, your muscles have nevertheless undergone strain and stretching during pregnancy.

Do practise Aswini Mudra (section 5, p. 106-7), doing steps 1, 2, and 8 first; later you can try steps 3 to 7. Practise it several times a day to help your bladder regain normal function, and to tighten the muscles of your pelvic floor.

Home again

For the first week or two at least after returning home, do avoid lifting, strenuous housework, and driving a vehicle. Remember: you've not only undergone major surgery, but you've also given birth. Your energy reserves will be lower than usual, and you need to spend a substantial part of each day resting and relaxing.

Sex and contraception

It's wise to wait until your cervix is closed before resuming sexual intercourse. *Check with your doctor.*

Here are some deterrents to mutually enjoyable sexual relationships:

● Disturbing noises (e.g. from the baby crying).

● Physical exhaustion (e.g. after a difficult day or a night without proper sleep).

● Fear of being less attractive than before (e.g. because of the incision scar).

● Fear of becoming pregnant again.

Discuss your concerns with your partner and encourage him to share his feelings with you. Don't feel compelled to resume previous sexual patterns. Strive for a greater mutual sharing and understanding. These will promote better communication and a closer, more mutually rewarding relationship.

Doctors generally prefer to insert an intrauterine contraceptive device (IUD) between 6 and 8 weeks after the baby's birth, so as to give the uterus a chance to involute properly and to avoid risk of infection. In the meantime, a condom may be used, along with suitable lubrication. (Sometimes, the emotional trauma of a caesarean experience can generate tension and diminish vaginal mucus.)

As already mentioned on page 56, breastfeeding is no guarantee of protection from pregnancy, and oral contraceptives are *not* recommended at this time.

There are now several 'natural' birth control methods which rely on fertility awareness rather than on chemical and mechanical aids. One of these is a computerized thermometer that records the woman's daily temperature and lets her know when it's safe to have intercourse. (There's a drop in basal body temperature about 24 hours before ovulation, followed by a sharp rise. The safe, infertile, period begins after the body temperature has remained elevated for at least 3 days.)

There are organizations to help people learn about natural birth control, and you may wish to get in touch with one of them for further information. It may also be useful to check with your library or bookstore for a book on the subject. Your local Family Planning or Well Woman clinic will be able to help.

Options

You may not have the final say in how your baby will be born. You do, however, have certain choices if you know that you're going to have a baby by caesarean section. Some of these options are:

- Requesting admission to hospital on the morning of surgery, rather than the day before, if this isn't absolutely necessary — provided that you prefer to do so.

- Requesting only partial pre-operative skin preparation, rather than the full routine which includes extensive shaving and an enema.

- Requesting information about medications you may be given.

- Being allowed to discuss a choice of anaesthesia.

- Asking for permission for your partner to be present at the birth, if circumstances permit this.

- Requesting a mirror through which to see the birth of your child.

- Asking to hold and nurse your baby as soon as possible after birth.

- Asking to nurse your baby while you're still in the recovery room.

- Requesting certain visiting privileges, such as few or no restrictions on visiting hours for the child's father, and permission for siblings to spend time with you.

- Asking to participate in a class especially designed for mothers who have given birth by caesarean section.

There are various caesarean support groups all over the country. Ask at your antenatal clinic or hospital for details.

Chapter 11

Hygiene Hints

The following are some points which you may wish to consider in conjunction with your personal hygiene during pregnancy and thereafter:

Care of the feet

Considering that the feet carry the weight of the body (and in pregnancy this weight is greater), we ought to spend more time than we do in looking after them. Chapter 6 gives some suggestions for exercising, strengthening and relaxing the feet.

During your pregnancy consider visiting a reputable chiropodist at least once, so that he or she may examine your feet to determine if they are perfectly healthy. If there are any corns, callouses or other abnormalities, these can be detected and suitably treated.

Select your shoes with the same care you give to choosing your maternity dresses, and buy shoes later in the day when a certain amount of swelling is not uncommon.

Care of the breasts

Breasts that are firm and well supported need little extra care. Bathing them with warm water is usually adequate, and the use of soap is not recommended. The darker appearance of the nipples in pregnancy is not an indication of accumulated dirt; it is nature's way of preparing them for the baby's vigorous sucking. Soap removes cells and secretions which help protect the skin of the nipples, and keep it acid and pliable. It destroys nature's protective barrier.

Any rubbing or massaging should be done strictly on your doctor's advice or as shown by a trained teacher at your prenatal class. Whatever the manipulation, it should be done gently. Be wary of applying ointments or lotions unless your doctor prescribes one. There should also be no pressure on breasts or nipples whether such pressure is manual or from a brassiere or other garment.

Care of the mouth and teeth

Visit your dentist at least once during your pregnancy, and have any conditions requiring treatment looked after. Infected gums or teeth are a septic focus where bacteria thrive and multiply. In pregnancy the body is already coping with the excretion of extra toxins; do not add to this burden.

The gums may be more sensitive at this time owing to an increased blood supply. If they tend to bleed, use a softer toothbrush. Rinsing the mouth with a weak solution of sea salt and warm water once or twice daily is beneficial because it is antiseptic and healing.

Do not brush the teeth from side to side. It causes the gums to recede, exposing part of the tooth structure called cementum. Cementum is very susceptible to wear and tear from abrasive toothpastes and powders, and to other factors which cause speedy decay.

Many dentists now recommend that the bristles of the toothbrush be held at an angle to the gum and allowed to penetrate slightly under the gum line. The brush is then vibrated firmly but gently for about 10 seconds per area until the whole mouth is covered. Gentle massage of the gums with clean forefinger and thumb each day is also a good habit which can contribute to their health. Use unwaxed dental floss at least once daily to disturb bacteria which help build up plaque.

Although not in widespread use, cleaning the tongue should be an essential part of oral hygiene. Try gently scraping it with an inverted teaspoon to remove accumulated deposits. Do this first thing in the morning before eating or drinking anything. You may be appalled at what you see! Imagine swallowing such deposits rather than removing them! A toothbrush is not suitable for this purpose; use a spoon or tongue scraper if you can find one. As you scrape the deposits, rinse away under running water and repeat the procedure. Cleaning the tongue daily will help eliminate bad breath and various stomach disorders.

Skin care

Skin can be at its loveliest during pregnancy, but it can also be problematic. For example, scars formed at this time tend to be darker and more noticeable than when you're not pregnant. This isn't because pregnant women scar more easily than non-pregnant women, but because their scars can be affected by changing levels of a hormone that intensifies pigmentation.

Freckles, moles or birthmarks can also darken. *Cloasma*, or the 'mask of pregnancy', may develop on the forehead, cheeks and elsewhere in the form of dark blotches.

Be especially careful when you shave, and don't pick at pimples; otherwise you may end up with unsightly marks.

Use soap sparingly; overuse of soaps can promote skin dryness and itching. It takes the oil glands about six hours to restore the skin's normal, protective acid-alkaline balance after a thorough cleansing with soap and water.

When venturing out into the sunshine, do use a moisturizing lotion with a sun protection factor (SPF) of 8 or more (SPF 15 or more in America) to help prevent damage from the sun's ultraviolet rays.

For a wealth of information on all aspects of skin care (and care of the hair and nails as well), you may wish to read my book entitled *Silky Smooth & Strong* (Thorsons, 1988).

Mental Health

Even though we may have a good general standard of hygiene, exercise regularly, eat, rest and relax adequately, if we are negative in our attitudes we cannot be truly healthy and happy. Yoga advocates the positive and denounces the negative. To be effective, yoga is not to be used merely as a superior physical culture system, but as a way of life that includes other factors such as correct deportment and positive attitudes. What are we if we are limber and energetic but selfish, devoid of compassion and constantly worrying about tomorrow? If you look in the Bible at St. Matthew's gospel, chapter 6, verses 25 to 34, you will see what Jesus Christ said with regard to having a positive mental attitude. It begins: 'Therefore I say unto you, Take no thought for [do not worry unduly about] your life, what ye shall eat, or what ye shall drink, nor yet for your body, what ye shall put on. Is not the life more than meat, and the body than raiment?' Jesus' advice here admonishes us not to let the negative emotions of fear and worry dominate our thoughts.

Try to cultivate a mental attitude which allows no room for worry, apprehension or fear, but one in which optimism and self-confidence replace those negative qualities.

By upgrading your general physical health through sound nutrition, proper exercise, correct breathing and good hygiene, you will be enhancing your mental health; by cultivating positive mental attitudes you will be enhancing your physical well-being. Let body and mind thus work together, with the help of yoga, to prepare you for becoming a truly healthy, happy, and serene woman, wife, and mother.

Chapter 12

Nutrition Notes

Good nutrition is an important part of prenatal care. A pregnant woman's diet should promote her own health, and at the same time provide correct nutritive material for the normal development of the foetus. Not only does proper nutrition maintain good health, but it also reduces the chances of complications in pregnancy. For those contemplating breastfeeding, an adequate diet is essential.

Pregnancy is a good time to become more informed about nutrition, and to initiate steps toward improving the nutritional status of yourself and your family. There are many informative books available at libraries and bookshops. Use them intelligently. May I offer two cautions? Firstly, do not at this time suddenly and drastically alter all your eating habits and the type of food to which you have been accustomed, perhaps for many years. It is too great an adjustment to ask of a body that is already having to make so many other adjustments. Use your common sense. Secondly, do not regard any one food item as a miracle food or over-indulge in it. No matter how many beneficial or miraculous properties may be attributed to certain foods, such foods are only part of the whole health picture. Equally important are such factors as good mental attitude, moderation, exercise, rest, relaxation, and correct breathing habits. They all play an important part in the satisfactory utilization of nutrients by the body.

The following represents some of the information which I have gathered from various nutritional works. I offer it to you for consideration, and for application wherever it may seem useful to you.

General

During pregnancy, vitamin and other supplements should be taken only with your doctor's approval. Some vitamin supplements do not include essential nutrients; an example of this is certain B vitamin supplements which do not contain choline. Choline is important in maintaining normal blood pressure, and works along with other vitamins and minerals to help prevent anaemia (deficiency of the red blood cells), a not uncommon condition among pregnant women. Vitamins and other nutrients must literally work together (they are synergistic in action) in order to be effective, and deficiency of one or more of them creates a demand by the body for those not provided. It would, therefore, seem wise to try to obtain, as far as possible, all the essential nutrients from natural sources where they are usually found in perfect balance.

In taking some dietary supplements, it is possible to take an overdose with toxic effects. Examples are the fat-soluble vitamins A and D.

Select your food with care. Try as far as possible to buy fresh fruits and vegetables, rather than canned or frozen. If you can be sure that they are organically grown, so much the better. Develop the habit of reading labels on jars, cans and packages. Choose only those with few or no preservatives or additives. Gradually substitute white flour with untreated wholewheat flour, reduce and eventually omit white sugar, using instead unpasteurized honey or other natural sweetener. Acquaint yourself with wholesome products such as many health food stores sell.

Prepare your food with love and care. Keep it simple. Serve it attractively, chew it properly, and eat it with a thankful heart.

Certain vitamins dissolve easily in water (the B complex and C). When preparing salad greens, for example, do not soak them in water. Rinse them quickly but thoroughly under cold, running water. Shake them dry and chill them quickly before cooking or eating raw. As far as possible, do not peel fruits and vegetables since precious minerals and vitamins lie just under the skins. Scrub vegetables under running water with a vegetable brush, and cook them with their skins intact.

Review your cooking methods and check your cooking utensils. Choose those which least destroy valuable nutrients. Get acquainted with the Chinese wok and the stir-fry method of cooking. There are many excellent cookbooks to enlighten you.

Eat moderately but adequately. Eating too little is perhaps as bad as eating too much. Chew your food thoroughly. The digestion of foods begins in the mouth through the action of the saliva. By chewing your food carefully, you are contributing to improved digestion. Finally, remember that individual needs and tolerances vary. What is right or adequate for one person may not be ideal for you.

Protein

Although protein requirements (as well, indeed, as those of all the other nutrients) are increased during pregnancy, the consumption of flesh foods as the major source of protein appears to be too high in industrialized nations such as ours. Alternative ways of obtaining sufficient first-class, usable protein

in the diet have been proposed by some writers on nutrition. In these days of high food costs, some of these alternatives may be worth looking into. For example, certain seeds and grains can be combined to produce good quality protein. A casserole of brown rice and beans would yield more grams of such protein than the rice eaten at one meal and the beans at another. Similarly, if you were to eat a peanut butter sandwich (made with wholewheat bread and a pure peanut butter) and drink a glass of milk at the same meal, you would be obtaining a complete protein. The same food items, however, taken separately at different meals, would not give the same value.

Vitamins from natural sources

Vitamin A

Parsley is an excellent source. Use handfuls of it in your cooking, rather than just a sprig as a garnish. Other sources are cod-liver oil, green-pigmented plants, yellow vegetables, peaches, yams, liver, butter.

Carrots, eaten raw, are good for massaging the gums. However, to receive the full vitamin content of what you eat, cook carrots lightly or extract their juice and sip it slowly.

Vitamin B complex

Many vitamins make up this group, and they should all be taken together daily. Taking only some of the B vitamins creates within the body a greater need for those not supplied. Since the milling and refining of whole grains deprive flour of the germ and the outer bran which are rich in the B vitamins, shun the use of white flour and use instead untreated wholewheat flour as a basic flour for making your own bread.

Other rich, natural sources of the vitamin B complex are yogurt (not because it contains these vitamins, but because it helps synthesize them in the intestines), brewer's yeast, blackstrap molasses, and liver.

Avoid using baking soda; it quickly destroys the thiamine in wholewheat flour and wheatgerm.

Drinking a great deal of coffee causes these vitamins to be washed from the body via the urine.

Egg white should not be used raw. When making an egg nog, for example, use only the yolk. It is thought that avidin, a substance present in egg white, combines with biotin (the 'mental health' vitamin) and prevents it from reaching the blood.

Be wary of buying milk in glass bottles. It may have been exposed to sunlight for many hours, in which case the riboflavin (vitamin B_2) will have been destroyed.

Folic acid (from 'foliage') is essential to help you utilize iron effectively. Together, these two nutrients help prevent anaemia which is not uncommon in pregnancy (see the section on iron). Folic acid is also needed in conjunction with calcium and vitamin K to help your blood clot satisfactorily and prevent excessive bleeding. For all these reasons your doctor will probably recommend that you eat a plentiful supply of green, leafy vegetables such as spinach, parsley, green leaf lettuce, turnip tops, mustard and cress, spring greens, and watercress. Try to eat these raw, as in a tossed salad, since cooking can destroy folic acid. Other sources are fresh mushrooms, soyabeans, sprouted grains, brewer's yeast, wheatgerm, liver, and kidney.

Vitamin C

When combined with substances known as the bioflavonoids, vitamin C is better utilized. The bioflavonoids are contained in the pulp and white part (just under the rind) of citrus fruits such as grapefruit, oranges and lemons. In addition to drinking fresh citrus juice, therefore, eat the fruit itself and include a small piece of the white part.

Vitamin D

Until recently, it was believed that adults had adequate reserves of vitamin D in their tissues, and that sunshine was the best source.

The most reliable source of this vitamin, however, is vitamin D-enriched milk. Butter, eggs and fish liver oils contain small amounts. Plant foods contain none.

Vitamin K

Called the anti-clotting vitamin, vitamin K is usually supplied adequately in foods and manufactured by the body in the intestines. However, since it does not pass readily through the placenta to the foetus, haemorrhage (bleeding) in newborn babies is not uncommon. For this reason, your doctor may give your baby an injection of vitamin K immediately after birth.

Please note that vitamin K is destroyed by antibiotics.

Minerals from natural sources

Iron

Iron is essential for the absorption of the oxygen we take in from the air we breathe, and for the transportation of this oxygen to every cell of the body. Transportation of oxygen to body cells is done through the haemoglobin (red colouring matter of the red blood cells), a deficiency of which leads to anaemia. Two signs and symptoms of iron deficiency anaemia are constant fatigue and shortness of breath.

The foetus is dependent on the pregnant woman for its iron supply, not only for its intrauterine survival, but also for its iron reserves during the first three months or so after birth. During these early months the baby's iron intake is low and poorly utilized.

The pregnant woman must, therefore, ensure an adequate supply of iron to maintain her own health and her baby's, and to allow some iron to be stored in its tissues.

Natural sources of iron are fresh fruit, apricots being the richest, green leafy vegetables (see folic acid), dried peas and beans, dried fruit (buy sun-dried), almonds, liver, egg yolk, wheatgerm, and blackstrap molasses.

Calcium

To help you keep calm and relaxed, make sure you are obtaining enough calcium. It is also essential for the formation of sound teeth and bones in the foetus, and is needed for proper blood circulation and clotting. To be assimilated, it must be combined *with the B vitamin complex, magnesium, vitamin D, phosphorus, and the unsaturated fatty acids.* Vitamin E in the diet must also be adequate so that the calcium is utilized by the bones and not laid down in the soft tissues.

Ideally, there should be no more than about twice the amount of phosphorus as calcium in the diet. When the phosphorus intake it too high, the surplus is excreted in the urine in the form of calcium salts, thus robbing the body of much needed calcium.

A good natural source of calcium is green leafy vegetables (preferably eaten raw). However, in spinach, for example, the oxalic acid present combines with the calcium to form an insoluble compound, calcium oxalate. Calcium oxalate prevents the calcium from being absorbed. Therefore, it is preferable to eat other green leafy vegetables such as the various leaf lettuces and alfalfa sprouts.

Other good sources of calcium are almonds, citrus fruits, dried figs, green vegetables (notably broccoli), milk and milk products, and sesame seeds.

The use of cocoa and chocolate appears to prevent the body from utilizing calcium. There is a substitute available (see next section) and it should be used if possible.

If you eat meat, increase your calcium supply by cooking meat that contains bone with tomatoes or a little apple cider vinegar. The acidity of these dissolves some of the bone calcium into the cooking liquid, all of which should be used.

Although skimmed milk is a good source of calcium, it ought not to be used as a substitute for fresh milk. In skimmed milk, the fat has been removed. In order for calcium to be absorbed into the blood, it must first be combined with fat. It then forms a soap in the intestines, and when this soap dissolves the calcium is released and passes into the blood. Therefore it is important to drink skimmed milk at a meal which contains some form of fat. If, however, you drink it between meals, take it with something that contains a little fat, such as a piece of crispbread and butter or peanut butter, or a few nuts eaten from the shell.

Sodium

Sodium is needed for normal heart action, it regulates body fluids, preserves a balance between calcium and phosphorus, and aids digestion. Natural sources are turnips, asparagus, cucumbers, courgettes (zucchini), marrow (squash), celery, carrots, string beans, beetroot (beets), oatmeal, coconut, figs, and raw egg yolk. With such rich natural sources of this mineral available, it is hardly necessary to add to foods the amount of salt many people do. Try cutting down on the amount of salt you add to your cooking, using sea salt instead of the usual commercial varieties.

Substitutes

Salt

Use dulse, also called sea lettuce. It is a dried, red seaweed used in certain northern countries. Put it in salad dressings, or use it as an alternative to lettuce in sandwiches, etc.

Kelp, another type of seaweed, may be used whole in soups. It imparts a pleasant, slightly salty flavour.

The following herbs may be used as salt substitutes in cooking. Experiment! Basil, savory, dill, celery seed and thyme.

Make the following 'herb salt' for use at the table: Powder (a small mortar and pestle will do), mix well then sift together equal parts of basil, savory, celery seed, sage and thyme.

Cocoa and chocolate

As noted earlier, calcium absorption appears to be inhibited by cocoa and chocolate. Carob, also known as 'St. John's Bread', does not have this effect. Made from the ground seed pods of a Mediterranean tree, it provides calcium, phosphorus and natural sugars and is low in starch and fat. Use carob powder in milkshakes and in baking biscuits and cakes.

Cornstarch

Instead of using this as a thickening agent for some Chinese-style dishes, soups, and gravies, use arrowroot flour which is high in minerals and not devitalized like cornstarch. Arrowroot is made from the root of a tropical American plant and sometimes is used in making rusks for infants.

Useful 'additives'

Non-instant powdered milk

Obtained from whole milk by a spray process, this white, fine milk powder has a mild odour and taste. Store it in a container with a tight-fitting lid to prevent any moisture absorption which could render it lumpy and disagreeable. It is superior to instant powdered milk and takes only two-thirds of a cup to reconstitute a litre of milk, whereas the instant variety requires one and one-third cups. Since it does not dissolve easily, however, you may need to mix it in a blender.

If you wish to cut down on your use of electricity, you may prefer to use this method: put one-quarter of a cup of warm or hot water into a tall, narrow container and add the powdered milk. Stir these ingredients together vigorously (a chopstick is useful), then add cold water for the rest of the volume, if you need cold milk.

Use non-instant powdered milk for fortifying beverages, cream soups and baked products, and for making yogurt.

Soya flour

Rich in an especially good quality protein, vitamins, calcium, magnesium, potassium and other minerals, as well as being low in starch, soya flour can add to the nutritive value of many foods. It is made from soya beans.

Use a small amount to thicken soups without altering their taste, and for every cup of other flour used in baking, use one tablespoon of soya flour to enrich and preserve the product.

Soya grits

Soya beans broken into very fine pieces are called soya grits. Simmer for about ten minutes in an equivalent amount of water and use to replace part of the meat in recipes such as meat loaf. Add a small amount to soups and stews during the last ten minutes of cooking to thicken and increase nutritive value.

Wheatgerm

When wheat is commercially milled and processed, the germ is usually discarded. The reason for this is that, if left in the milled flour, the germ becomes rancid very quickly and shortens the shelf life of the product. The germ, however, contains many valuable nutrients such as iron, the B vitamins and vitamin E. Buy it from a shop where they refrigerate it (store it at home in the same way), and add it to cereal, fruit, and in making breads and cookies. The reason for refrigerating wheatgerm is to prevent its becoming rancid; if it does it can destroy vitamin E.

Sunflower seeds

Sunflower seeds contain, in almost perfectly balanced amounts, perhaps all the essential nutrients. Use them in making your own cereal (muesli or granola), biscuits or cookies, and as a topping on fruit, or eat them raw or lightly toasted.

Brewer's yeast

Do not confuse this yeast with the one used as a leavening agent in baking. Brewer's yeast is available in powdered or flake form and is high in minerals and vitamins, notably the B vitamins. Vegetarians, who sometimes find it difficult to obtain an adequate amount of vitamin B_{12} from other foods, find brewer's yeast indispensable. Add it to fruit or vegetable juices, and to cakes, biscuits, cookies and other baked goods to increase their nutritive value.

You would be wise to use a fortified yeast so as not to risk upsetting the calcium/phosphorus ratio in your diet.

Yogurt

Yogurt helps the body synthesize the B vitamin complex in the intestines. Avoid the fruit-flavoured kind sold commercially. Usually it contains refined sugar and chemical additives. Make your own and use it as a superb quick breakfast, a sustaining snack, a dessert either on its own or mixed with fruit salad, a topping for baked potato, or as a base for pancakes and waffles.

Sprouts

Sprouts are germinating seeds at the peak of their activity, at which stage they are more nutritious than either the original seed or the plant they ultimately produce. They are an excellent source of the B vitamins, vitamins C and E, and protein. Mung beans (a variety of soyabean) sprouted can be used in Chinese style dishes, soups, omelettes and salads. Wheat sprouts can be chopped and used instead of part of the flour in making bread. Sprouted lentils can be used in much the same way as mung bean sprouts. Alfalfa sprouts, perhaps the most nutritious of all, should be eaten raw in sandwiches, salads, in blender drinks, or by themselves.

Natural laxatives

The following natural foods are useful for their mild laxative action; there is no need to resort to commercial laxatives, especially those with a mineral oil base. Such laxatives can leach from the body the fat soluble vitamins A, D, E, and K.

Honey — unpasteurized, from bees which were not fed sugar.

Wheatgerm, blackstrap molasses, yogurt, figs, raisins and prune juice, and natural bran (not to be confused with 'all bran' or other processed cereals).

Natural sedatives

Try to draw upon your own natural resources to obtain sound sleep. See chapter 6 for suggestions on sleep.

A deficiency of B vitamins in the diet may contribute to insomnia. If you suspect this, try to rectify it by increasing your intake of foods known to be rich in these nutrients.

Insomnia is also sometimes related to a low calcium level in the blood. The following bedtime drinks will provide some calcium and may be helpful in inducing restful sleep:

- Whole milk, fortified with non-instant powdered milk, with a little honey.

- Blend one cup milk, one egg yolk, one teaspoon brewer's yeast, one teaspoon carob powder and one teaspoon honey.

- Peppermint tea with or without a little honey.

- A tea made as follows: Steep in boiling water for about ten minutes (use a non-metal utensil) equal parts of scullcap, valerian and catnip or mint. Let cool and add a little honey or use plain.

All the above drinks should be sipped slowly at bedtime. A warm bath before retiring is relaxing, and may be effective in promoting sleep. The water should be about 35°C (95°F).

Natural aids to labour

Substitute red raspberry leaf tea for the ordinary variety. It contains *fragarine*, a property which is thought to contribute to an easy labour by helping relax the uterine muscles.

Spikenard, long used by native Indian women, is credited with being useful in making labour short and easy.

Contraindications

Ferrous sulphate as an iron supplement is strictly forbidden in pregnancy because it destroys vitamin E rapidly. The destruction of this vitamin can cause miscarriage.

Do not take baking soda in water to relieve heartburn or indigestion. The sodium content is too high.

Chapter 13

Post Partum

The post partum period is the time immediately following the birth of your baby (from the Latin *post* meaning 'after' and *partum* having borne'). The first six weeks after childbirth are known as the 'puerperium' (from the Latin *puer* meaning 'child' and *parere* 'to bring forth'). It is during the puerperium that the reproductive organs are rapidly returning to the nonpregnant state, the most marked changes occurring in the breasts, abdomen, and pelvic organs.

The breasts

The breasts do not alter noticeably in appearance during the first two or three days after the baby is born. During this time they secrete 'colostrum', a thin, somewhat yellow fluid, abundant in nutrients. Between the third and fourth days approximately, colostrum begins to be replaced by milk. The breasts then become engorged, but please be reassured that this engorgement and the discomforts which it produces will disappear in a day or so.

The following are thought to help increase milk supply; whole grain cereals, especially oatmeal, and plenty of water. For those who will not be nursing and wish to decrease their milk flow naturally, reducing the daily fluid intake and drinking sage tea instead of ordinary tea are considered useful.

The abdomen

The abdominal wall has been stretched immensely during the previous nine months. Immediately after childbirth, when the tension from the enlarged uterus is removed, the skin of the abdomen becomes flabby. With proper care the abdominal muscles should approach their original tone in two or three months.

Most women appear to recover from the exertion of labour quickly, and feel well generally. When one considers the many changes which the body has undergone during the nine or so months of pregnancy, it is remarkable how rapid is the return to the nonpregnant state.

Walking

Walking is one of the best forms of exercise after having a baby. With your doctor's permission, walk around your room to help re-establish normal blood circulation. The weight of the uterus on the pelvic blood vessels during pregnancy will have slowed down the circulation a great deal. Later on, weather permitting, take baby for a daily 'walk' in a stroller. During these walks, stand tall maintaining the good posture which, hopefully, you acquired during the previous months. Breathe slowly and deeply, and practise the Rhythmic or Walking Breath (section 8) for part of the walk.

Rest and relaxation

Make sure you obtain adequate rest and relaxation, especially if you are breastfeeding. Successful lactation is dependent in part on the quality of these.

Pain from episiotomy

Several forms of treatment are used to promote rapid healing of an episiotomy. Co-operate with your doctor in this matter. To help yourself practise tightening and relaxing the muscles of your pelvic floor (Aswini Mudra, step 8, section 5) as soon as your doctor says you can. It will help improve the blood supply to this area, giving a measure of relief from congestion which may be one underlying cause of pain. Continue your breathing and relaxation techniques. They will help you overcome the pain.

'Fifth day blues'

Some women become depressed about the fifth day following childbirth. There are many theories as to the cause or causes. Whatever they may be, however, you can gain some relief by practising the Alternate Nostril Breath (section 8) and relaxation techniques as described in section 6.

Exercise

Please *check with your doctor* as you did pre-natally, before engaging in any form of exercise. There may be reasons why he or she may not wish you to exercise in the early days after childbirth. The nature of your labour will determine largely the type of activity in which you may indulge and how soon to start. Immediately after the birth, muscles and ligaments which support the uterus are lax. They have been stretched enormously during pregnancy and labour. The uterus can, therefore, be displaced easily until such time as its supporting structures regain normal tone. If permitted to exercise, start with very gentle body movements, done slowly and carefully as always, gradually working toward more challenging poses.

The following is a guide only:

First week after birth

1. Stretch the whole body from head to toe (variation of the Standing Pose, section 4). You may now point the toes away from you.

2. Do slow, deep abdominal breathing, done about three times daily. Contract the abdomen on exhalation (refer to chapter 8). You may do this while lying in bed.

3. Rotate the ankles, first clockwise then counterclockwise, an equal number of times, to help re-establish normal blood circulation in the legs. You may do this while sitting on the edge of the bed with your legs dangling.

4. Walk around the room or house. Hold yourself tall. Breathe comfortably.

5. The Pelvic Tilt (section 3).

6. Aswini Mudra (section 5). Make sure the bladder is empty. If you had an episiotomy, ask your doctor how soon you can re-commence this exercise. In the early post-natal days there may not be much sensation in the pelvic floor, and control may be poor. However, keep trying, concentrating keenly all the time.

7. Alternate Nostril Breath (section 8). This breath may be a boon during moments of depression (e.g. 'fifth-day blues') or frustration (e.g. while trying to establish successful breastfeeding).

8. Deep relaxation in the supine position (the

Sponge, section 6). You may do this in bed.

9. Deep relaxation in the prone position (p.131).

Second week after birth

Continue doing the poses you have been practising during the first postnatal week, and add the following:

1. Gently begin to tone and strengthen the abdominal muscles by lying flat in bed (no pillow), legs outstretched in front and arms relaxed at your sides, palms down. Bend your knees just enough to allow you to place the soles of your feet flat on the bed. They should not be too near the buttocks. Exhaling, raise only the head and look down at your abdomen which you should feel tighten. Hold for a second then lower the head as you inhale. Repeat. Relax. As the abdominal muscles become stronger, omit repetition but prolong the holding period, breathing normally as you do so.

2. Raised Leg Posture (section 1). Try the first and second variations to begin with.

3. The Knee Press (section 3).

4. The Mountain Posture (section 8).

Six weeks after birth

Your doctor will probably wish to see you about six weeks after your baby's birth. You will be examined to determine essentially whether your uterus has returned to its normal condition, has not been displaced, and your perineum has healed satisfactorily. All being well, you may ask permission to resume gradually the exercises you did prenatally, and to add new ones. You will find the four postures described on pages 132-137 particularly beneficial.

When you select poses for your daily yoga session, try to include one each of the following:

Technique	Example
Breathing exercise	The Mountain Posture (section 8)
Forward bend	The Cat Stretch (Fig. 62)
Backward bend	The Cat Stretch (Fig. 63)
Sideways bend	The Side Leg Raise (section 9)
Twisting movement	The Spinal Twist (section 3)
Pelvic floor exercise	Aswini Mudra (section 5)
Bust exercise	The Chest Expander (section 7)
Leg exercise	The Cat Stretch (Fig. 63) The Side Leg Raise (section 9)
Complete relaxation	The Sponge (section 6)

An inverted and a balancing pose would complete your session ideally. Since, however, I did not include such poses in this book, you may refer to some of the yoga books available in local libraries and bookstores.

Exercise Sections

Limbering Up

The Leg Flop

Benefits

- Loosens the ankle, knee, and hip joints.
- Stretches and tones the adductor muscles running along the inner thighs.

Technique:

1. Sit with the legs outstretched in front and comfortably separated. You may place your hands on the floor beside you for support and balance.

2. Bend the right leg (you may use your hands) bringing the sole of the foot opposite the left thigh, and letting the knee fall outward.

3. Bend the left leg as you did the right and place the sole of the left foot against the sole of the right one.

4. Keeping the body erect but not rigid, and relaxing the facial muscles, hold the feet together by clasping the hands around them (Fig. 9). Take a few slow, deep breaths and then pull the feet as close to the pubic area as comfortable. Alternatively, pull the feet close to you and then place the hands on the floor behind the hips, fingers pointing away from you. Straighten arms and spine. Later in pregnancy when the abdomen is quite large, this may prove a more convenient arrangement.

5. Alternately lower and raise the knees (indicated by the direction of the arrows in Fig. 9) in a sort of flapping motion, like a bird flapping its wings. Repeat the movements several times, incorporating a comfortable breathing rhythm.

6. Relax, breathing normally.

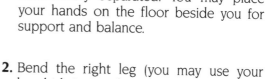

Fig. 9   *The Leg Flop. The arrows indicate the up and down movement of the knees.*

The Raised Leg Posture
(Alternate Leg Raise)

Benefits:

- Limbers, strengthens and tones the ankles and legs.

- Warms up, strengthens and tones the muscles of the back and abdomen.

Technique:

1. Lie on your back with the legs outstretched in front and fairly close together. Arms are relaxed alongside the body, with the palms turned downward (Fig. 10).

2. Press the small of the back against the floor to reduce the spinal arch there, to protect the back and abdominal muscles from possible strain, and to help you

Fig. 10 *Preparing for the Raised Leg Posture.*

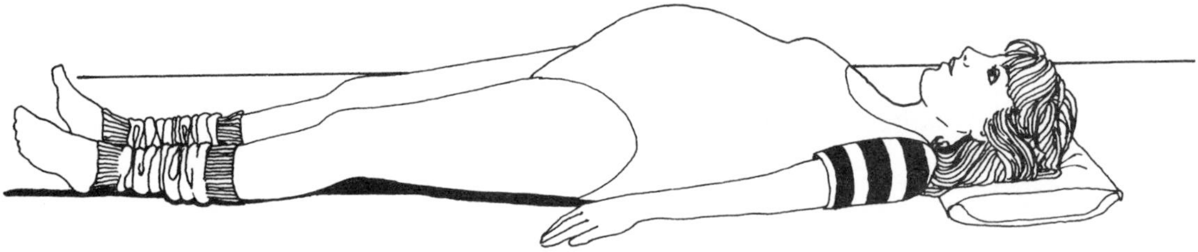

Fig. 11 *The completed Raised Leg Posture (Alternate Leg Raise).*

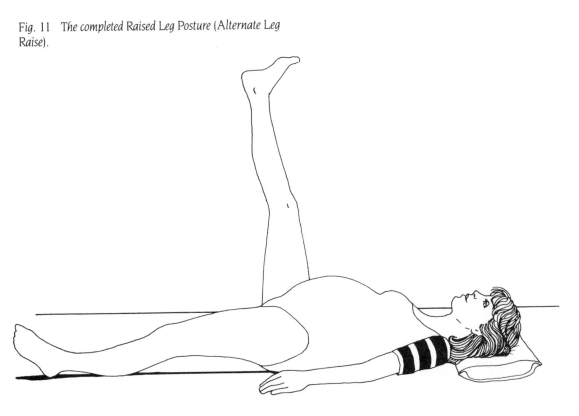

80

control the leg movements to follow. Your knees may bend slightly as you do this, but this is perfectly all right if comfortable.

3. Locking the right knee, that is, keeping it straight, pull the toes toward you as you simultaneously push the heel away from you. With the leg in this position you are now ready to raise it. Keep the left leg relaxed.

4. Slowly raise the right leg off the floor (Fig. 11). Some people find it easier to exhale as the leg is raised; others prefer to inhale. Experiment to find what is more comfortable for you. When you have raised the leg as far as comfort permits, hold the position for a few seconds, breathing as normally as possible.

5. Slowly and carefully lower the leg, inhaling or exhaling as preferred. Relax, breathing normally.

6. Repeat steps 2 to 5, raising the left leg this time, and keeping the right one relaxed on the floor.

Variation 1:

1. Lie down as depicted in Fig. 10. Bend the right leg at the knee and bring it toward the chest, allowing it to fall slightly outward rather than directly onto the abdomen. Do this on an exhalation.

2. Slowly and carefully straighten the leg as you inhale. Hold this position, breathing normally.

3. Bend the leg at the knee as you exhale, and lower it to the floor as you inhale. Relax, breathing normally.

4. Repeat steps 1 to 3, raising the left leg this time.

5. Perform these movements about three times with each leg.

Variation 2:

1. Lie as depicted in Fig. 10.

2. Bend the right leg just enough to place the sole of the foot flat on the floor.

3. Slowly and carefully raise the left leg, incorporating rhythmical breathing. Hold the raised leg position for a few seconds, breathing as normally as possible. Lower the leg carefully. Relax. Repeat twice. Relax.

4. Repeat steps 2 and 3, raising the right leg this time.

The Cat Pose

See section 3, Figs. 19 and 20 only. This asana is excellent for keeping the spine supple as well as strengthening the back and abdomen.

The Sitting Postures

The Disciple (or Student) Posture

Technique:

1. Sit comfortably erect with the legs out-stretched in front of you. To begin with, you may place your hands on the floor beside or behind you for support.

2. Bend your right leg at the knee, and with the help of your hands, place the sole of the foot against the inner surface of the opposite thigh (Fig. 12). If this is too difficult, place it against the knee or other part of the leg that is easiest to reach.

3. Place your hands over respective knees or in any other comfortable position, and make sure that the whole body, facial muscles included, is at ease.

4. After a while, change the position of the legs so that the right is outstretched and the left bent.

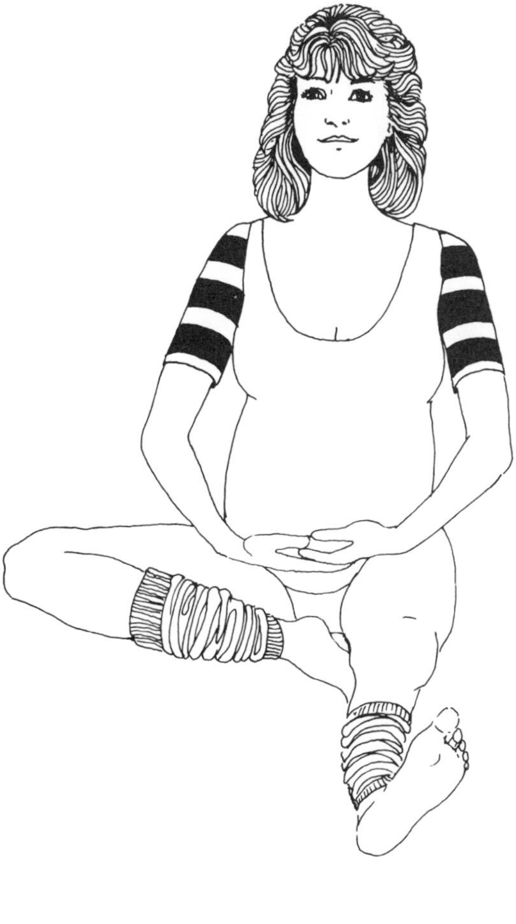

The Easy Pose

When sitting in this pose you are said also to be sitting 'tailor fashion' because the position beings into play the sartorius or tailor muscles which lie across the thighs, from about the front of the hip bones to what we know as the shin bones. These muscles are

Fig. 12 The Disciple (Student) Posture.

the ones used in bending the legs and turning them inward, movements which will be involved in this pose.

Technique 1:

1. Sit comfortably erect with the legs outstretched.

2. Cross the legs at the ankles and, supporting yourself with the hands on the floor beside you, draw the crossed legs close to the body, as near to the pubic area as possible. Relax the legs to permit the knees to fall outward (Fig. 13).

3. Sit in this position with your hands resting quietly on your knees, or upturned, one on top of the other, on the lap. Check to see that all parts of your body not directly involved in the movements are relaxed.

Technique 2:

1. Sit with the legs outstretched in front and, if necessary, place the hands on the floor beside you for support.

2. Bend the right leg and place the foot under the left thigh.

3. Bend the left leg and place the foot under the bent right leg (Fig. 13).

4. Place your hands over respective knees or, upturning them, place one in the other on your lap and let them rest quietly.

5. Keep the body erect without being rigid, and relax the facial muscles.

Note:

If the knees are not close to the floor at first, do not be disheartened. As the joints become more flexible and the ligaments more elastic, the knees will come near the floor.

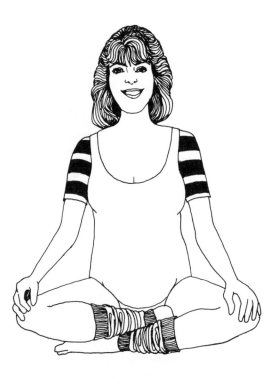

Fig. 13. *The Easy Pose (sitting tailor fashion).*

The Perfect Posture (or Pose of an Adept)

Technique:

1. Sit comfortably erect with the legs outstretched in front.

2. Bend the right leg and place the sole of the foot against the left thigh as far up as possible.

3. Bend the left leg and slowly and carefully place the foot in the crease formed by the right thigh and calf (Fig. 14). Ideally, the left heel should touch the pubic bone.

4. Place the hands over respective knees or rest them, upturned, quietly in the lap.

5. After a while, change the position of the legs so that the right leg is now uppermost.

2. Begin to lower your body very slowly as if to sit on your heels. In so doing, you may find that you will have to incline slightly forward to avoid losing balance. When you have lowered yourself to the point where it is possible to touch the floor beside you, begin to use your hands to assist you in balancing, and also (at the beginning anyway) to share in bearing some of the body's weight. Slowly try to sit upon your heels, but if for the present this is impossible, or your feet cannot bear the weight of your body, then use your hands as suggested.

3. If you have managed to sit on your heels (Fig. 15), place the palms of your hands over respective knees, and sit in this manner for a few seconds to begin with; hold the position longer after you are

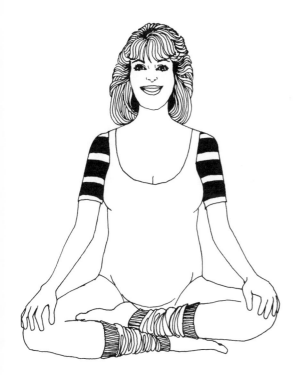

Fig. 14. *The Perfect Posture* (*Pose of an Adept*).

Note:

As in the other cross-legged postions, the knees should ultimately come near to or touch the ground. However, do not force them to do so. Be patient, persevere, and in time they will.

The Firm Posture (Japanese Sitting Position)

This is also known as the Diamond Posture, the Thunderbolt Posture, and the Hardy Posture.

Technique:

1. Kneel down with the legs together and the body erect but not rigid. Let the feet point straight backward.

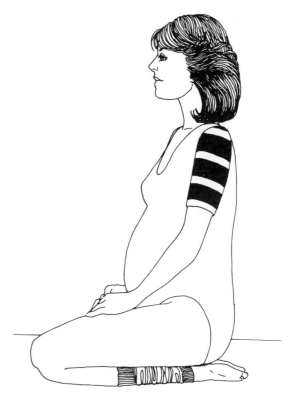

Fig. 15 *The Firm Posture* (*Japanese Sitting Position*).

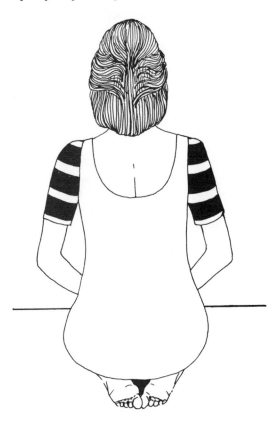

Fig. 16   *Variation of the Firm Posture.*

accustomed to the posture. Practise slow, deep, regular breathing.

Variation:

Let the heels fall apart but keep the toes together. Sit in the space formed by the parted heels (Fig. 16).

Suggestion:

If you find the weight of your body on your heels too great at first, place a flat cushion or folded towel between buttocks and heels.

The Sitting Warrior

Whereas most of the sitting postures described are not as a rule recommended for use by those who suffer from varicose veins, as already explained, this pose may be practised by anyone for short or long periods.

In addition to the other benefits derived from practising the sitting postures, the Sitting Warrior is excellent for relieving tired, aching feet and legs. It is also probably the only posture that can safely be used immediately after a heavy meal, as it helps relieve any discomfort that may be felt in the stomach.

Technique:

1. Keeping the body erect but not rigid, kneel down with the knees together but the feet

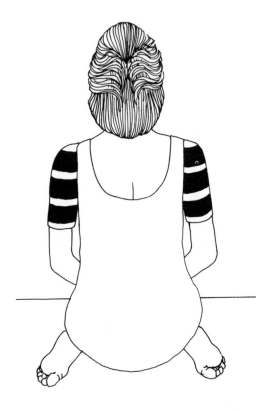

Fig. 17   *The Sitting Warrior position.*

as wide apart as possible, and certainly at least the width of your bottom.

2. Slowly lower your body, using your hands to assist you wherever necessary, and try to sit on the floor between the parted feet (Fig. 17). Place your hands over respective knees, or let them lie, one on the other, in the lap.

3. Remain in the pose for as long as you can with absolute comfort, breathing slowly, deeply and evenly.

4. Very slowly and with control come out of the position by reversing the steps for going into the pose. Use your hands to help you. No strain whatever must be placed upon the back.

Dynamic variation:

Follow steps 1 and 2. When you can lower yourself no farther, let your hands take most of your weight and use them to help you raise yourself up again. Repeat these movements, alternately lowering and raising the body. This improves the blood circulation in the legs.

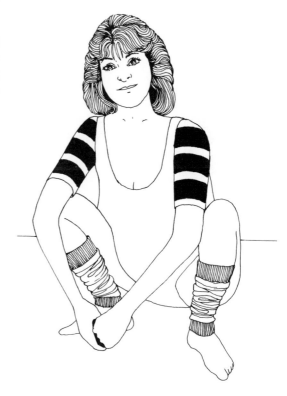

Fig. 18   The Squatting Pose.

The Squatting Pose

Caution: This pose, in its static form, is *not* recommended for use by persons who have varicose veins. Such persons may, however, practise the dynamic variation.

Benefits:

● The squatting position is the most natural and most efficient one both for childbirth and for emptying the bowel. During labour you may be placed in a position which is, in fact, a modified squatting position, where your legs are wide apart and your feet supported. In the squatting position, the muscles of the pelvic floor are

stretched and the pelvic diameter is enlarged. It stands to reason then, that habitual use of this posture will be good preparation for ease of birth.

● Squatting helps make the muscles of the pelvic floor more elastic. This is thought to be of value in shortening that period of labour just before the birth.

● Squatting reduces the curve of the spine at the small of the back (this curve may be exaggerated by pregnancy). Consequently, relief is afforded the muscles and ligaments supporting the spine. There is less pressure on the discs between the bones that make up the spine. As a result, the back is strengthened and relaxed, and back discomforts kept to a minimum.

● Squatting is marvellous for helping correct constipation.

- Squatting is excellent for strengthening the ankles and feet.

- It tones and strengthens the abdominal muscles.

- It has been said that the occurrence of breech births (where the bottom rather than the head is born first) is rare among primitive people, and attributed in part to the fact that these people squat a great deal.

- The incidence of varicose veins, piles, and uterine prolapse appears to be low among people who habitually squat.

Technique:

1. Stand with your legs comfortably apart, taking the body's weight evenly on both feet.

2. Bend the knees slowly, keeping the feet firmly planted on the ground and slowly lower your body until your buttocks come as near as comfortably possible to the heels. When you begin to go downward, incline your body somewhat forward, keeping your arms outstretched, and using them to help you keep your balance. Exhale as you lower yourself. Keep your feet sufficiently wide apart to accommodate your abdomen when you finally manage to sit on your heels. Let your arms hang forward loosely between your knees, or arrange them in whatever way you find most convenient, perhaps hanging over your knees with your upper arms resting on them (Fig. 18).

3. Hold this position for as long as comfortable, breathing slowly and rhythmically. If you find it easier to place your hands on the floor beside you to help with support and balance please do so. You must be comfortable.

4. Inclining slightly forward and using the arms to help with balance, slowly raise the buttocks from the heels and come to a standing position while inhaling. Loosely shake your arms and legs to help them relax.

Dynamic variation:

Stand with legs apart and arms at the sides. Inhaling, slowly raise the arms sideways to shoulder level as you simultaneously raise yourself onto your toes. Do not take chances with losing your balance. If necessary, hold on to a stable piece of furniture with one hand as you raise yourself.

Exhale slowly while lowering your arms and body to the squatting position described in step 2 of the Squatting Pose. Without holding the postion, come up again on tiptoe, and repeat these up and down movements a few times. Relax.

Alternately lowering and raising the body in this manner contracts and stretches the muscles of the legs. The blood vessels of the legs are gently massaged by the muscular movements, and the flow of blood improved. Pressure on the walls of the blood vessels from a sluggish blood flow is temporarily relieved.

Strengthening the Back and Abdomen

The Cat Pose (pelvic rocking)

Benefits:

- When the spine is parallel to the floor, the internal organs fall freely forward with consequent relief to certain internal ligaments.

- In the upright position, the enlarging uterus compresses pelvic blood vessels and impedes blood circulation to the legs and kidneys. It exerts a tremendous pull on the ligaments which attack the uterus to the spine, weakening the lower back. The 'all fours' position temporarily relieves these conditions.

Fig. 19. The 'table' position in preparation for the Cat Pose (pelvic rocking).

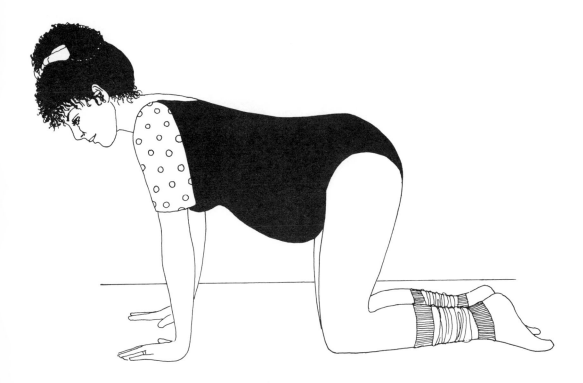

- The spine is exercised and the spinal muscles and ligaments toned and strengthened.

- The abdominal muscles are toned and strengthened to support the weight of the enlarging uterus more effectively.

Technique:

1. Kneel down on 'all fours'. In this position the knees and the palms of the hands are in contact with the floor. The arms and thighs are perpendicular to it, the arms being about the width of the shoulders apart, and the legs comfortably separated. In this position the back is fairly level, like a table on four legs. Since some people's arms and legs are not proportionate, the back may not be absolutely level. Be comfortable. (See Fig. 19).

2. Exhaling, slowly lower your head, press down on your hands and hunch your shoulders. At the same time tuck your bottom well under to tilt your pelvis slightly forward (Fig. 20). These movements should be performed slowly and smoothly to last the length of your exhalation.

3. Hold the position for a few seconds, breathing normally.

4. Inhaling, slowly allow your body to relax into the starting position described in step 1. The natural inward curvature of the spine should not be accentuated.

5. Sit back on your heels or use some other comfortable position in which to relax, breathing normally.

Fig. 20   *The completed Cat Pose.*

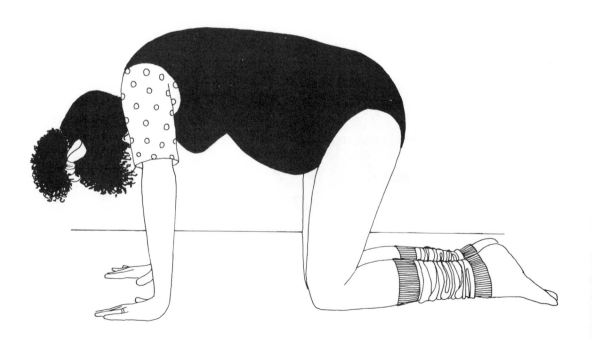

Variation:

Get into the 'all fours' position and move your hips from side to side, like an animal wagging its tail. Keep the shoulders 'facing' forward and let the action proceed from the waist.

Suggestions:

You may use the 'all fours' position when dusting lower parts of furniture, wiping something which has been spilt on the floor, to amuse a small child, or to search for a tiny object. Pause for a few seconds and practise steps 2 to 4.

Performed at bedtime, this posture helps counteract the effects of gravity on your body in its upright position during the day. You will feel more relaxed and probably sleep better after doing it a few times.

Note well:

Figure 21 depicts a movement, normally part of the Cat Pose, which is the opposite of that described in step 2. Because it accentuates the concave arch of the lower back, it is not recommended during pregnancy as it may be conducive to backache.

The Knee Press (Wind-relieving Pose)

Benefits:

● Strengthens the abdominal muscles.

● Strengthens the muscles of the neck, shoulders and back.

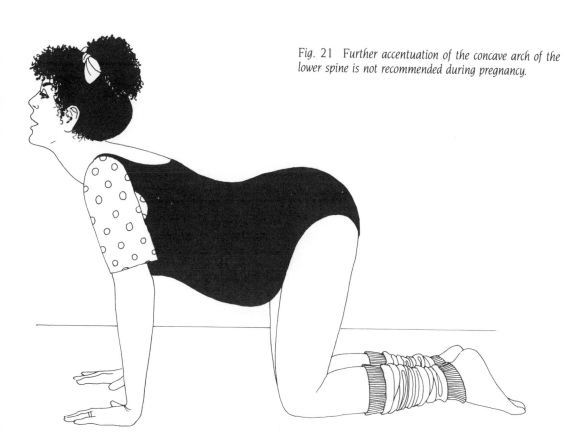

Fig. 21 Further accentuation of the concave arch of the lower spine is not recommended during pregnancy.

- Relieves back strain and backache.

- Helps dispel gas from the stomach and intestines.

- During labour a modification of this pose is usually used when the baby is about to be born. It decreases the space in the abdominal cavity and, together with the breath, exerts pressure on the diaphragm to help push the baby out.

- Improves elimination of waste matter from the body through the bladder and bowel.

Technique:

1. Lie on the back, legs outstretched in front and arms alongside the body. Keep the small of the back pressed to the floor as much as possible.

2. Exhaling, slowly bend the right leg and bring it as close as you can toward the body. If the abdomen is already quite large you will find that you will need to let the knee fall somewhat outward as you draw it toward you. Now clasp your hands around the bent leg (Fig. 22). Keep the shoulders relaxed.

3. Hold the position for a few seconds breathing normally.

4. Inhaling, slowly release the hold on the leg and gradually lower it to the floor. Keep the small of the back pressed to the floor.

5. Relax for a few seconds, breathing normally.

6. Repeat steps 2 to 5, bending the left leg this time.

Variation 1:

1. Follow step 2.

2. Bend your head forward and try to touch the bent knee with it (Fig. 23).

3. Hold the position for a few seconds, breathing as normally as you can.

4. Release the hold on the leg and carefully lower arms, head, then leg to the floor. Relax, breathing normally.

Fig. 22   Knee Press (Wind-relieving Pose).

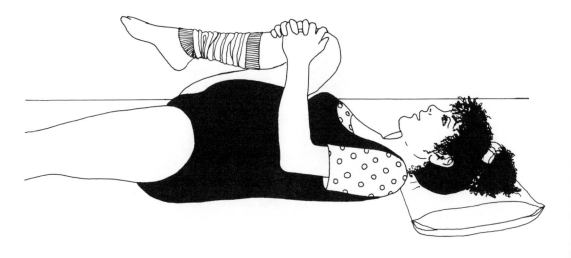

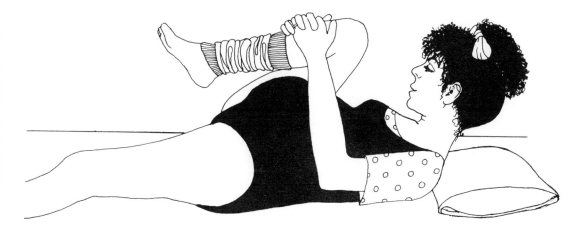

Fig. 23   Knee Press — Variation 1.

Variation 2:

1. Lie as described in step 1.

2. Bend one leg, then the other, resting the soles of the feet on the floor. Bring both legs toward the body while exhaling. The legs should be sufficiently separated to accommodate the abdomen without putting pressure on it. Clasp each knee with the corresponding hand, keeping the elbows well out to help maintain the separation of the legs and allow the chest to expand adequately. Now you will be able

Fig. 24   Knee Press — Variation 2.

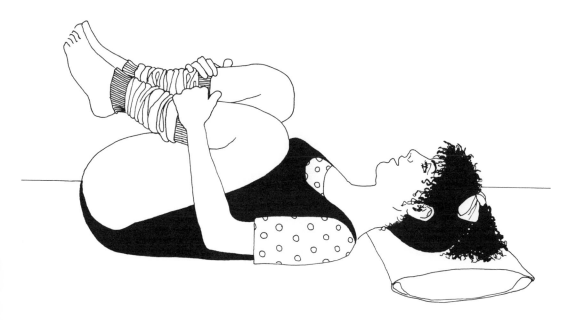

to breathe deeply (Fig. 24). Relax your shoulders.

3. Hold the position for a few seconds, breathing evenly and as deeply as possible.

4. Slowly release the hold on the legs and lower them, one at a time, to the floor. Keep the small of the back pressed to the floor. Relax, breathing normally.

Variation 3:

1. Follow steps 1 and 2 of Variation 2.

2. Keeping the legs in this position, bend the head forward and try to touch the chest with the chin (Fig. 25). Keep the shoulders as relaxed as possible.

3. Hold the position, breathing as deeply as comfort permits, for a few seconds.

4. Release the hold on each leg in turn and carefully lower it to the floor. Relax, breathing normally.

Notes:

If you feel more comfortable maintaining the hold on the bent leg or legs by placing your hands underneath rather than over them, please do so.

In the latter part of pregnancy you may find it more comfortable to sit with several pillows behind you in order to practise the postures just described. Arrange your prop so that your back is at about a 45-degree angle to the floor.

Fig. 25 Knee Press — Variation 3.

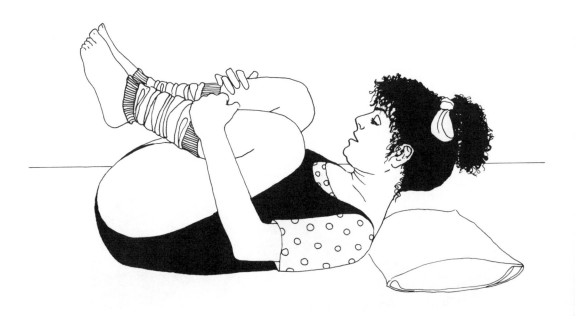

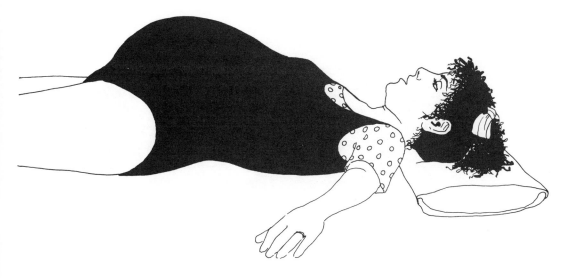

Fig. 26 The normal spinal arch of the lower back.

The Pelvic Tilt

Benefits:

- Strengthens the lower back and helps relieve fatigue, aches, and pain in that area.
- Tones and strengthens the abdominal muscles.

Technique:

1. Lie on your back with legs outstretched in front and arms beside you.

2. Slide your hands under your waist and note the arch in the back (Fig. 26). The idea is to remove that arch temporarily. Return your arms to your side.

3. Establish a comfortable breathing rhythm. Now on an exhalation, slowly and carefully press the small of your back to the floor to remove the arch (Fig. 27). You should feel your abdominal muscles tighten and your pelvic tilt slightly upward. Hold the position as long as the exhalation lasts.

4. Relax as you inhale.

Note:

You may find that, especially at the beginning, you need to bend your legs a little and perhaps tighten your buttocks the better to tilt the pelvis.

Variation:

Lie on your back and bend your legs so that the soles of the feet rest comfortably on the floor. Exhaling, carefully press the small of the back to the floor and let the pelvis tilt slightly upward. Hold as long as exhalation lasts. Relax as you inhale.

Suggestions:

Practise pelvis tilting several times daily by standing against a wall and trying to press the small of the back into it as you exhale. Hold. Relax. When you are in an elevator, try to stand against the side of it and do the same thing.

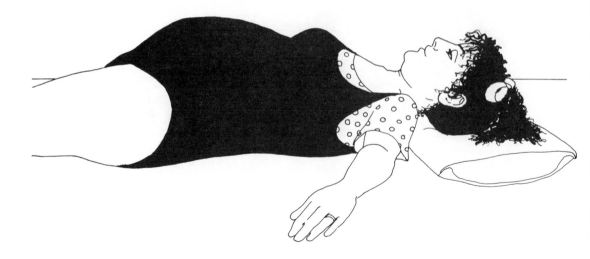

Fig. 27 *The Pelvic Tilt temporarily reduces the lower spinal arch.*

The Back Push Up (Bridge or Reverse Arch)

Fig. 28 *Preparing for the Back Push Up (Bridge or Reverse Arch).*

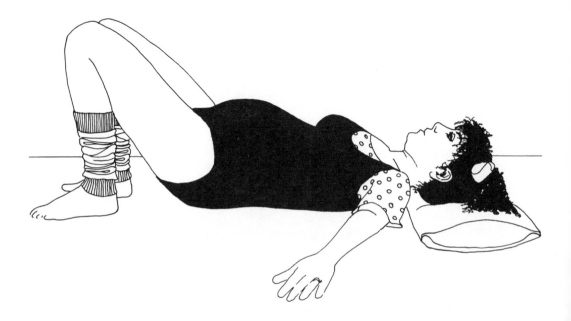

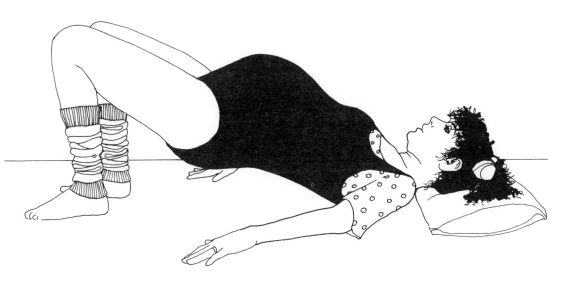

Fig. 29 Completed Back Push Up.

Benefits:

● As for the Pelvic Tilt.

Technique:

1. Lie on your back with legs outstretched in front and arms alongside the body, palms down.

2. Bend the legs and pull the feet as close to the buttocks as comfortable, keeping the soles firmly on the floor and the legs as close together as you can (Fig. 28).

3. Keeping soles, arms and body from the shoulders upward firmly in contact with the floor, raise the buttocks carefully, slowly, and as high as you can without strain while inhaling (Fig. 29). You may find it helpful to press knees, thighs and buttocks firmly together to assist with raising the hips.

4. Hold the position, breathing normally.

5. Slowly reverse the order of the movements

while exhaling, and return to the position described in step 1. If you visualize these movements as a slow unrolling of the spine, starting with the vertebrae between the shoulderblades, and working toward the bottom, it may help you come out of the posture in the most beneficial way. Done in this manner, the spine is gently but effectively massaged. When you reach the small of the back, press it firmly into the floor.

6. Lying outstretched or with knees bent and brought close to the body (see Fig. 28, p.96), relax, breathing normally.

Spinal Twist (Simplified)

Benefits:

● The Spinal Twist exercises the usually weak transverse and oblique muscles of the abdomen.

97

- The Spinal Twist contributes to the flexibility of the spine.

- The nervous system is toned because of the large number of nerves along the spinal column receiving stimulation.

- Helps combat constipation.

- Aids digestion.

Technique:

1. Sit in the Firm Posture (Fig. 15, p.85).

2. Bring the left hand across the front of the body and tuck the fingers in the cleft formed by the right calf and thigh. You now have leverage to help with the subsequent twisting action of the trunk. You may place your right hand on the floor beside you for support and balance (Fig. 30).

3. Having established your balance, slowly

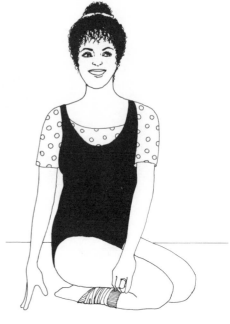

Fig. 30   *Preparing for the Spinal Twist (Simplified).*

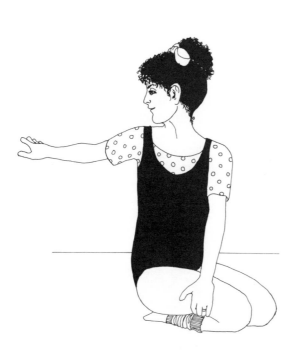

Fig. 31   *Movement toward the Spinal Twist — head and eyes follow the backward sweep of the arm.*

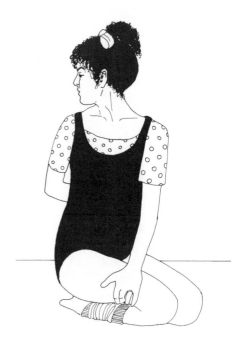

Fig. 32   *The completed Spinal Twist.*

raise your right hand off the floor to about shoulder level, turning the palm backward. Inhale as you do this.

4. Exhaling now, press backward with the outstretched arm, simultaneously turning your eyes, head and shoulders to follow its movement (Fig. 31). The arm movement is reminiscent of a swimming stroke.

5. When you can turn no farther, bend your elbow and place your hand against your spine, somewhere near the small of the back, with the palm turned away from the body (Fig. 32).

6. Maintain this body twist for a few seconds as you breathe comfortably.

7. Let the right hand fall and, inhaling, slowly turn your body to face forward. Rest your hands quietly on your knees and relax, breathing normally.

8. Repeat steps 2 to 7, twisting to the left this time (substitute 'right' for 'left' in the instructions, and vice versa).

Variation:

People with varicose veins may welcome an opportunity to practise the Spinal Twist without having to sit on the heels. Sit naturally erect on a chair. Your feet should rest firmly on the floor, toes relaxed, and you should face directly forward. Establish a comfortable breathing pattern. Now on an exhalation, slowly and carefully turn your body from the waist upward to the left, keeping the pelvis 'facing' forward and the bottom firmly on the chair. When you can twist no farther, hold on to the back of the chair with the left hand, and to your left thigh or side of the chair with your right hand. Look over your left shoulder. Maintain the position for a few seconds, breathing as comfortably as possible. Slowly and carefully come out of the position in reverse order while inhaling, and relax, breathing normally. Repeat the twist to the right side.

The Sideways Swing (Atlas Posture)

Benefits:

● Tones and strengthens the little used transverse and oblique abdominal muscles.

● Contributes to spinal flexibility.

Technique:

1. Sit upright with both legs bent to the left of the body.

2. Inhaling, raise your arms upward and interlace your fingers over year head. The upper arms should be alongside your ears.

3. Exhaling, slowly and carefully incline your body sideways in the direction of the legs (Fig. 33).

4. Hold the position for two or three seconds, breathing normally.

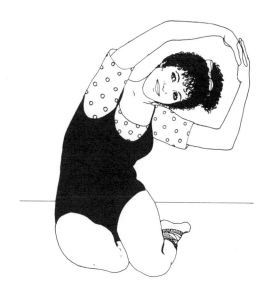

Fig. 33 The Sideways Swing (Atlas Posture).

5. Return to the upright position, again slowly and carefully, as you inhale. Rest, breathing comfortably.

6. Move the legs to the right side and repeat steps 2 to 5, bending to the right this time. Relax, breathing normally.

Posture and Body Mechanics

Standing Pose

Benefits:

- Helps you acquire an appreciation of correct stance where the body's weight is evenly distributed between the feet.
- Cultivating the habit of standing tall will help reduce harmful stress.
- The upward stretch of the arms will help you gain better chest expansion and improved lung capacity. It will facilitate deeper breathing and thereby improve aeration of the lungs.
- The muscles on the chest, abdomen and pelvis are toned.
- Blood circulation to all the internal organs is improved.

Note:

Stretching upward to one's comfortable limit will not cause the umbilical cord to slip around the baby's neck and strangle it. This is an 'old wives' tale' which is ridiculous, and like other such tales, should not be entertained. A relaxed mind is every bit as important to a healthy pregnancy as a relaxed body.

Technique:

1. Stand tall, but comfortably so, with feet

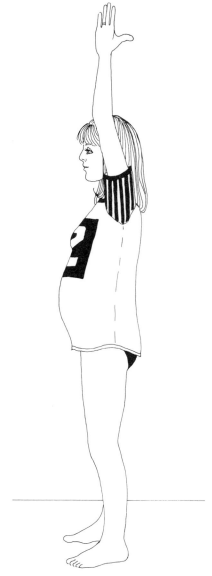

Fig. 34 A *Standing Pose.*

either touching each other or slightly apart. Please do not try to simulate a military stance; this only increases the curve of the lower back and produces fatigue. The arms are at the sides with the shoulders relaxed, and the chin is not jutting forward. This would produce tension in the neck.

2. The weight of the body should be equally and evenly distributed along the entire soles of the feet. Keep the toes relaxed.

3. Bring the arms slowly upward from alongside the body, inhaling as you do so. Keep the upper arms near the ears and try to bring the palms together over your head (Fig. 34).

4. Hold this position for a few seconds, breathing normally.

5. Slowly lower the arms as you exhale. Relax.

Variation:

The same principle of an all-over stretch may be applied while lying on the back. Inhaling, bring the arms upward and slowly and carefully stretch your body to its full length. Bring the toes toward the body while pushing away with the heels. Hold this position for a few seconds, breathing normally. Lower the arms and relax the feet and legs as you exhale. Relax.

The Pelvis and Pelvic Care

The Star Posture

The Star Posture is so called because the completed pose, when seen from above, resembles a star — the head, the bent elbows, and the bent knees forming five points.

Caution:

Since this pose involves a forward bending movement, use it with discretion after about the fourth month of pregnancy. Although the parted thighs allow a space to accommodate the enlarging abdomen, physiques do differ and you should adapt movements to suit your own body. You should feel no undesirable pressure on the abdomen.

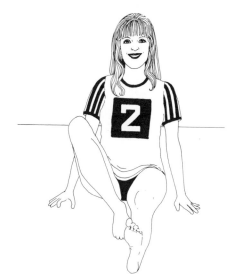

Fig. 35 *Preparing for the Star Posture — establish the correct distance between feet and body.*

Benefits:

- Prepares the pelvic floor for ease of birth by stretching, toning, and relaxing the muscles in that area.

- Helps keep the spine flexibile, thus contributing to reduction of back fatigue and backache.

- Helps to keep the hip and knee joints flexible.

- Aids digestion.

Technique:

1. Sit comfortably erect with the legs outstretched in front. If you wish, you may place the hands on the floor beside you for support, to begin with. Take a few comfortable breaths and compose yourself.

2. Bend the right leg at the knee and place the sole of the foot flat on the floor opposite the inside of the left knee (Fig. 35). This will establish the correct distance from foot to body. Maintain this distance throughout the exercise.

3. Bend the left leg as you did the right, and place the soles of the feet together (Fig. 36).

4. Clasp the hands firmly around the feet. Inhale. Now exhaling slowly, bend forward

103

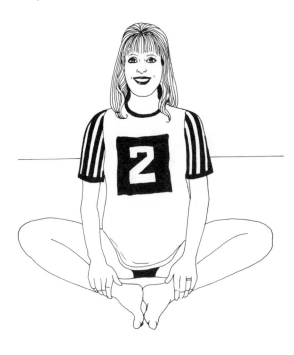

Fig. 36 *Preparing for the Star Posture — soles of the feet are together.*

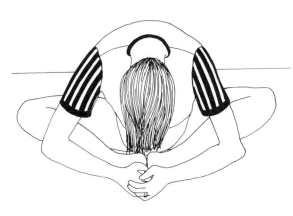

Fig. 37 *The completed Star Posture.*

carefully. Continue the forward bending movement slowly, gradually, and with control, trying to bring your face toward your feet (Fig. 37). Do not strain. Note that the elbows flare outward and are kept outside

of the legs. What matters is the effort because, however feeble it may appear to you, it is still producing results. Persevere. When you have reached your comfortable limit, hold the position for a second or two (more if absolutely comfortable), breathing as normally as possible during the holding period.

5. Very slowly come up to your initial sitting position as you inhale. Straighten your legs, place your hands on the floor beside you and relax, breathing comfortably. Did you remember to keep your facial muscles relaxed?

6. After performing a forward bending movement it is usual to offset it with a backward bend, or at least a backward inclination of the body. With your hands just behind the hips, on the floor, and fingers pointing away from the body, press downward on the hands, carefully bend your head backward, pointing the chin upward and giving the neck a delightful stretch. If you can, slightly lift the buttocks of the floor. Hold the position for a couple of seconds and then release. Relax. Incorporate breathing as follows: inhale as you bend the head backward, breathe as normally as possible as you hold the position, exhale as you release the hold, and breathe normally as you relax.

The Star Posture may also be followed by the Pelvic Tilt or the Back Push Up (section 3).

The Knee and Thigh Stretch

Benefits:

● Provides intense stretching of the deep and superficial muscles which run along the inner thighs (adductor muscles). This in turn tones muscles and ligaments within the pelvis, promoting the health of the entire pelvic area.

- Prepares your muscles for being in the labour position without resulting strain.

- The ankle, knee, and hips joints are exercised and kept strong and supple.

- A rich supply of blood is brought to the back and abdomen, and the kidneys and bladder benefit. It has been said that Indian cobblers, who habitually sit in this position, do not usually suffer from urinary disorders.

- Sitting in this position for a short while each day will discourage the development of varicose veins.

- Regular practice of the posture can help reduce the intensity of labour pains.

Technique:

1. Sit on the floor, with your body comfortably erect and legs outstretched in front. To begin with, you may place your hands beside you on the floor for support and balance. Relax your body, including your facial muscles. Establish comfortable respiration.

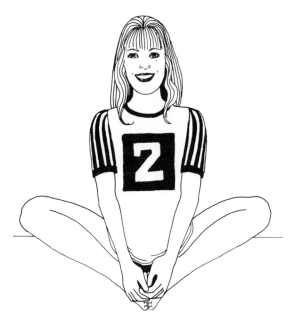

Fig. 38 Preparing for the Knee and Thigh Stretch. Bring the feet as close to the body as comfortable.

2. Bend the right knee, and, using your hands, bring the sole of the foot against the inside of the left thigh as far up as possible.

3. Take hold of the left foot and place the sole against the right sole. Try not to lose your balance; use your hands to help stabilize you, if necessary.

4. Maintaining a comfortably erect position of the trunk from now on, and remembering to keep your face relaxed, place your hands around the feet and pull them as close to the body as comfortably possible (Fig. 38). Inhale slowly while performing this movement.

5. When your feet are as close to you as possible, continue holding on to them and try to press the knees toward the floor as you exhale (Fig. 39). Do not tighten your

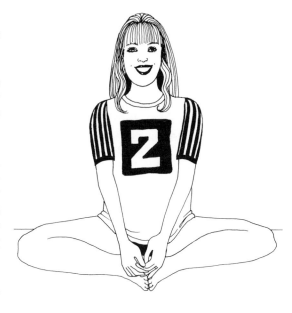

Fig. 39 The completed Knee and Thigh Stretch.

facial muscles; keep them relaxed. You may find that if you pull upward on the feet while pressing downward with the knees you may be more successful in getting the knees near the floor. If at first they cannot get near the floor, do not despair. They eventually will as your joints become limber and the muscles and ligaments more elastic with regular practice.

6. When you have reached your ultimate comfortable stretch, hold the position only for as long as you can with ease, breathing normally.

7. Inhaling, slowly and carefully allow the knees to come upward, remove the hands from the feet, and gradually straighten the legs. You may place your hands beside you on the floor for support, and move your legs about by alternately pulling and pushing the heels along the floor to help them relax. Breathe comfortably.

Variation of step 5:

If your abdomen is quite large already, instead of holding on to the feet as depicted in Fig. 38, place the hands on the floor behind the hips, fingers pointing away from you. Straighten the arms and back and, pressing the feet together, carefully lower the knees to the floor as you exhale. Hold the position for a second or two, breathing as normally as possible and keeping the facial muscles relaxed. Inhaling, let the knees come upward slowly. Relax, breathing normally.

Aswini Mudra

The numerous benefits of this technique have already been outlined. It is suggested that, before attempting it, you empty your bladder and, if possible, your bowel also.

Note well:

This is a fairly powerful exercise, so do not repeat it too often at any one time. Instead, do it again two or three times during the course of the day.

Technique:

1. Sit in any comfortable position, lie down or stand, and remember to keep your facial muscles as relaxed as possible.

2. Inhale and exhale slowly, deeply, and evenly for a few seconds.

3. Inhale. Now while slowly *exhaling*, contract your anus by pulling inward and upward. If you think in terms of trying to prevent a bowel movement, this may help you appreciate the sensation you want to feel. Hold the contraction for as long as your exhalation lasts with comfort.

4. Inhale slowly as you release the contraction. Relax, breathing normally.
   In the female, the rectum (of which the anus is the opening), the vagina (birth canal), and the bladder (of which the urethra is the opening) lie one behind the other, so that their respective muscular walls adjoin. By contracting the anal muscles, the urethra and vagina are also being exercised. The three openings are part of one large muscle, yet it is possible to contract and release each opening with little or no movement from the others. Although this is not at first easy, patience, concentration (and visualization of the desired ultimate effect), as well as consistent practice will bring progress toward achieving an excellent control of these muscles individually, and of the pelvic floor as a whole. Acquiring such control will be invaluable to you both during childbirth and afterward.

5. Now try to contract only the vaginal muscles as you *exhale* slowly, and hold the

contraction for the length of your exhalation. Relax your facial muscles.

6. Slowly release the contraction as you inhale. Relax, breathing normally.

7. Now try to focus your attention on the opening through which urine is passed (the urethra). This is much more difficult to control, but it is possible, and perseverance is worthwhile. To gain an appreciation of the desired sensation, try the following: Next time you go to the toilet, start to pass urine. Part of the way through, stop the flow temporarily and hold this interruption for a few seconds. In so doing you are tightening the sphincter muscle of your urethra as well as its muscular walls. Now continue the flow of urine. Again interrupt it for a few seconds, if possible. Finally finish the flow. The sensations which you felt during the pauses you made should give you some idea of what you should experience during the actual exercise. Remember that you *exhale* when contracting the muscles, and inhale when releasing them. Try not to tighten either the anus or vagina when trying to contract the urethra. This requires much concentration. To help concentration, try to visualize your experiment in interrupting the flow of urine and the sensations experienced then. Do not be disheartened if you are not successful at first. Keep trying. One day, surprisingly, you will have gained this subtle control!

8. Finally (and this should be the easiest), inhale, *exhale* slowly while contracting the whole pelvic floor (all three orifices — anus, vagina and urethra). Hold the contraction for as long as the exhalation lasts.

Slowly release the muscles as you inhale. Relax while breathing normally. Did you remember to relax your face?

Suggestions:

The cross-legged sitting positions and squatting, described in section 2, are beneficial to the health of the pelvic floor. Any movement which stretches the muscles running along the inner thighs is beneficial. Two ways in which you may incorporate such movements into your daily activities are:

1. Walk up stairs two or three at a time, depending on how steep they are and how long your legs. Use the handrail for support. Inhale as you lift the leg, exhale as you step forward. Take the weight on the entire surface of the sole of the foot.

2. When in the garden or elsewhere in the open, hold on to a fence or tree trunk, and do forward lunging movements as follows: Stand erect with the legs wide apart. Step forward with the right foot. Exhaling, bend the right knee and slowly shift your weight onto the entire sole of the right foot. The right knee projects beyond the foot, and the left leg drags behind you. Do not arch the small of your back inward. Keep the back straight but relaxed. Hold the position, breathing normally, then inhaling, return to your starting position. Repeat the forward lunging movement with the left leg.

Lunging movements can be done indoors. Hold onto the back of a sturdy chair or other suitable piece of furniture for support.

Tension and Relaxation

The Sponge (Corpse Posture or the Pose of Deep Relaxation)

The Sanskrit word for this pose is *Savasana*. It denotes that the body is supine with the limbs lying passively at full length, in much the same way as a corpse. It has therefore come to be known as the Corpse Posture — not a very pretty name, but one which is truly descriptive. More pleasant sounding names are given above, the Sponge implying that the body is open to suggestion, absorbing all that it is taught in the technique — and it does have to be taught how to relax completely!

Deep and complete relaxation is not achieved by simply flopping down somewhere. It is a neuromuscular (referring to nerves and muscles) skill which has to be learnt. The ability to release tension from a muscle requires concentration in much the same way as it does to contract it actively.

The Sponge is not easy to master. It requires much patience and may take as long as twenty minutes or even more at first attempt to execute correctly. However, you will eventually be able to do it quite quickly in just a matter of a few minutes. Do persevere — it is a technique hailed by many medical people for the innumerable benefits it bestows.

Practise the Sponge as many times during the day as you need, and always at the end of your daily yoga session. Once mastered, the technique may be applied even when you are sitting or semi-recumbent.

Benefits:

The following are only some of the innumerable benefits of the Sponge:

- Done in the evening, it is excellent for promoting sound sleep. It is a superb natural tranquilizer.
- Gives deep relaxation to nerves and muscles, helping eliminate all forms of tension.
- Helps keep the blood pressure within normal limits.
- Useful in learning to conserve energy.
- Contributes to poise and vitality.

Technique 1:

Use this technique at first. After you have mastered it, you may prefer to use technique 2. Although it is not necessary to contract a muscle group actively in order to relax it, you are asked in this technique to do so, observing the feeling of tension in that part of the body as you hold the contraction for two or three seconds. You are then asked to release the contraction, again observing how that part of the body feels. This provides a means of comparison between the way a muscle group or part of the body feels in a state of tension, and the way it feels during a state of complete relaxation. When the ability to differentiate between these two states has been perfected through regular practice of the technique, you will be able to relax any part of your body at will, without first going through the motions of alternate contraction and relaxation. You can then use technique 2 on a regular basis, if you wish.

Here is yet another chance to involve your partner. Ask him to read the instructions to you the first couple of times, or until you know them by heart. This will leave your mind free to concentrate fully on what you are about to do.

The following points should be observed during practice of the technique:

● Establish and maintain a comfortable breathing rhythm throughout. Do not hold your breath at any time.

● Relax all parts of the body which are not being actively contracted. Concentrate fully on the part being contracted.

● After you have contracted a muscle group, hold the contraction for two or three seconds, studying carefully what is happening to that part of the body and how it feels. Remember this feeling.

● After releasing the contraction, again study carefully what has happened to that part of the body. Note how it feels, and compare this feeling with that experienced when the muscles were contracted. Remember it. Let us begin now.

1. Lie on your back with one or more pillows under your head, and wherever else needed for comfort, support and/or easing of pressure. You must be very comfortable. The legs are sufficiently separated to ensure that no tension is encouraged in the hip area. Keep the knees slightly flexed and let the feet fall outward. The arms are well away from the body, palms upturned in an attitude of total surrender. Fingers curl inward slightly. If the arms are too close to the body the shoulders will be pushed upward, inviting tension. The eyes are closed or at least without expression. Do not let the chin protrude as this will result in tension in the lower jaw and neck. Breathe easily. (See Fig. 40).

2. Push the heels away from the body, bringing the outspread toes toward you. Remember to keep all other parts of the body limp, and breathe comfortably. Hold. Release.

3. Press the back of the knees firmly against the surface on which you are lying. Tighten the knee-caps. Concentrate on the muscles of the lower leg. Hold. Release.

4. Contract the thigh muscles as tightly as possible. Hold. Release.

Fig. 40 *Basic body position for the Sponge (Corpse Posture or Pose of Deep Relaxation).*

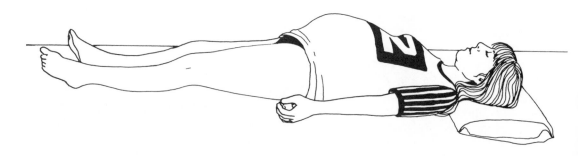

5. Squeeze the buttocks together very tightly. Hold. Release.

6. Exhale as you slowly and firmly press the small of your back against the surface on which you are lying. Tighten your abdominal muscles. Hold for as long as exhalation lasts. Release as you inhale. Rest, breathing normally.

7. Inhale deeply as you squeeze the shoulderblades together. Do not lift the arms. Hold, breathing normally. Concentrate on the tension of the muscles across the chest. Release as you exhale. Rest, breathing normally.

8. Bring the shoulders upward as if to touch the ears. Hold. Release.

9. Bending the head backward and keeping the lips together but not compressed, push the chin upward. Hold. Release.

10. Bend your head forward, tucking the chin well in. Hold. Release.

11. Raise the eyebrows, squeezing the forehead to form horizontal wrinkles. Hold. Release.

12. Squeeze the eyebrows together tightly to form a frown. Hold. Release.

13. Squeeze the eyes to close them tightly. Hold. Release.

14. Opening the eyes, slowly and deliberately circle them first clockwise then counterclockwise. This is to enable you to recognize tension in the eyeballs. Close the eyes.

15. Curl your tongue far back against the roof of your mouth. Hold. Release.

16. With lips together but not compressed, clench the teeth. Hold. Release.

17. Open your mouth widely as if to say 'a-ah'. Hold. Release.

18. Stretch the lips from ear to ear in your widest possible smile. Hold. Release.

19. Bring the corners of your mouth downward in an effort to frown. Hold. Release.

20. Make the lips round as if to say 'boot', or as if to whistle. Hold. Release.

21. Now focus your attention on your arms and hands. Turn the palms down. Bend the wrists backward, fingers stiffened and outspread. Hold. Release.

22. Turn the palms upward, fingers relaxed. Bring the hands toward the forearms. Hold. Release.

23. Stiffen the arms and make tight fists. Bending them now at the elbows, bring the fists toward the shoulders. Hold. Release.

24. Turn the palms up. Stiffening the arms, push away from you with the hands. Hold. Release.

25. Whenever thoughts enter your mind, do not try to send them away forcefully as this will produce tension. Let them drift inward but do not try to expand them; simply let them drift onward and outward.

26. Focus your attention now on your breathing. With each incoming breath feel the intake of lightness, energy and balance. With each exhalation feel the outflow of fatigue poisons, negative feelings and imbalance. Slow down your respirations; make them deeper and smoother. Feel peace and tranquility enfold you.
Remain like this for several minutes, after which prepare to get up slowly.

27. Gently stretch your limbs as your body dictates. Make your movements leisurely. Do not point your toes too vigorously. Delight in all these stretching movements, then slowly turn on to your side. With the help of your arms and hands, return to an upright position (see Fig. 30, p.98).

Note:

Intense pointing of the toes away from the body is not a good idea in pregnancy, as it seems to contribute to leg cramps. If you experience such a cramp, try pushing the heel away from the body, bringing the toes toward you.

Technique 2:

In this technique, you are dispensing with actively contracting muscle groups prior to releasing them. Presumably you now fully appreciate how a group of muscles or part of the body feels in a fully relaxed state.

1. Lie as in step 1 of technique 1 (Fig. 40).

2. Mentally going over the body from top to toe, concentrate in turn on each group of muscles, or you may care to think of it as each part of the body. Give patient, loving suggestion to that part to go loose and limp, to let go of tension, and to relax. With each inhalation, feel life-force entering your body; with each exhalation an outflow of fatigue and tension. If at any point your mind wanders, gently persuade it back to concentration.

3. Continue thus until you have covered every part of your body. The facial muscles are very important. Pay special attention to the lower jaw, tongue, throat and eyelids. They hold subtle forms of tension which, if not released, are an obstacle to complete relaxation.

4. Breathe slowly and evenly. Do not encourage thoughts or forcefully try to shut your mind to their entry. Simply let them drift in and out. Remain in this state of total relaxation for several minutes.

5. Arise slowly and carefully after some

gentle stretching movements, feeling refreshed and revitalized.

Note:

If light disturbs you, tie a dark scarf around your eyes, making sure that the knot does not put pressure on the head or face.

The Lion

This asana, frightful though it may appear, is excellent for releasing tension from the facial muscles and those of the throat. Teachers of singing and elocution will confirm that in many people the lower jaw and throat are exceedingly tense, and among the most difficult parts of the body to relax.

Benefits:

● Tones the facial muscles and is therefore beautifying. Pregnancy is a time when you can be radiant, and many women are.

● Contributes to the relaxation of the pelvic floor and indeed to the whole body.

● Brings a rich supply of blood to the throat area. Can improve the condition of a sore throat. If you feel a sore throat threatening, the Lion can help prevent it from developing.

● Helps improve the quality of the voice.

Technique:

1. Sit on the heels as in the Firm Posture (Fig. 15, p.85) with the palms of the hands over the knees. For those of you who cannot use this position, the pose may be done in any other suitable one.

2. Inhale. Exhale slowly and at the same time open the eyes and mouth as widely as possible. Very slowly stick out the tongue as far as it will go, but do not gag. Feel the

Palming

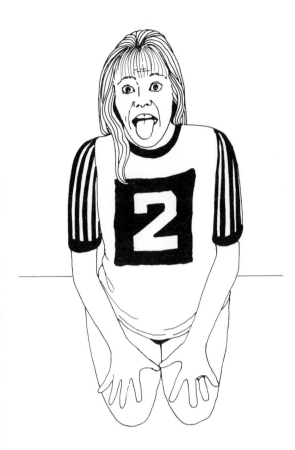

Fig. 41   The Lion — look as fierce as you can!

muscles of the face and throat become taut. Stiffen the arms and spread out the fingers. The idea is to look as fierce as possible (Fig. 41).

3. Hold the pose for as long as your exhalation lasts with absolute comfort, then slowly relax the tongue, facial muscles, arms and hands. Do these reverse movements while inhaling. Relax, breathing normally. Close your eyes and visualize all tension dissolving from your face.

Benefits:

● Diminishes fatigue from the eyes, face and whole body.

● Aids concentration.

● Helps bring a sparkle to the eyes.

Technique:

1. Rest the elbows comfortably on the table or desk at which you are working, or squat and rest them on your knees if you can. You may even practise palming in a lying position.

2. First, rub the palms of the hands together vigorously to warm and charge them with electricity. It is believed that this electricity imparts to the eyes a natural vitality.

3. Now place the palms gently over closed eyes so as to exclude all light. The fingers rest lightly on the forehead, those of one hand being close to those of the other (Fig. 42). No pressure must be exerted on the eyeballs. Try to concentrate on relaxing the eyelids. It is not easy to do, but keep on trying since much tension lodges in these muscles.

4. Remain in this position for a minute or more, breathing slowly, deeply and regularly.

5. Keep your eyes closed and repeat steps 2 to 4 if you wish. If not, proceed to step 6.

6. Separate your fingers and open your eyes to allow a slow re-introduction of light. Gradually lower your hands, and shake them to get rid of any tension. Blink your eyes a few times.

Practise palming as many times each day as you wish, in or out of doors.

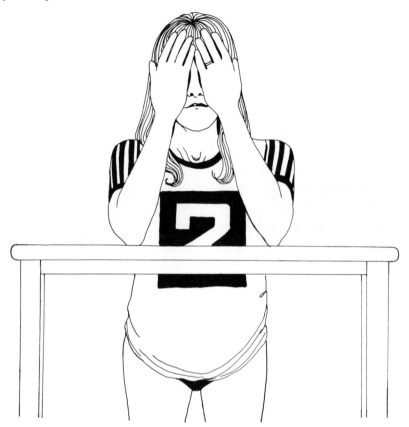

Fig. 42 *Palming — a welcome rest for tired eyes.*

Head Rolls

Benefits:

- Breaks up calcium deposits which have accumulated between the bones of the neck, reducing stiffness in this area.

- Releases tension from the lower jaw, throat and upper back, areas which are great storehouses of tension.

Technique:

1. Sit comfortably erect, keeping the arms, hands and shoulders relaxed throughout the movements. You may close your eyes if you wish. Close your mouth, but do not tighten your lips; keep your teeth unclenched. Relax your facial muscles.

2. Let the head fall forward loosely and hang there limply for a few seconds. Breathe comfortably. Raise the head.

3. Let the head fall backward slowly and hang there limply for a few seconds. Breathe comfortably. Raise the head.

4. Incline the head to the right shoulder. Hold. Breathe comfortably. Raise the head.

5. Incline the head to the left shoulder. Hold. Breathe comfortably. Raise the head.

6. Maintaining your comfortable breathing rhythm, slowly and loosely rotate the head two or three times in a clockwise direction, then in a counterclockwise one the same number of times. Relax.

The Blade

Benefits:

- Releases tension harboured between the shoulderblades, thereby contributing to the relaxation of the whole body.

- Helps tone and strengthen the underlying muscular supports of the enlarging breasts, reducing the chances of a drooping bustline later on.

Technique:

1. Choose a comfortable sitting position such as the Firm Posture (Fig. 15, p.85). If using a chair, sit sideways so that the back of it does not hinder your movements.

2. Inhaling, raise the arms sideways to shoulder level, then bend them at the elbows to bring them inward across the front of the chest. The fingertips should touch lightly (Fig. 43).

3. Exhale. Inhaling slowly, gradually push backward with the upper arms, trying to bring the shoulderblades together with a steady, squeezing motion. In so doing, the fingertips will part (Fig. 44).

4. When you can go no farther, hold the position for a few seconds, breathing normally.

5. Exhaling, slowly release the hold and let your arms fall to your sides. Relax the

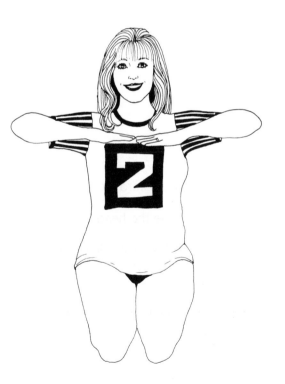

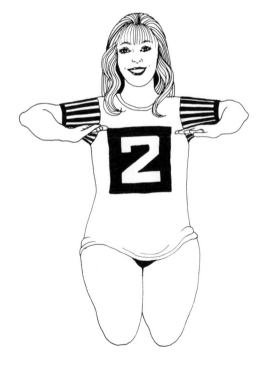

Fig. 43   Preparing for the Blade.

Fig. 44   The completed Blade.

shoulders by shrugging them a few times, and the hands by shaking them loosely.

Legs Against the Wall

Benefits:

● Relieves tired and swollen feet. By elevating the legs, the return flow of blood to the heart is aided, and the valves of the large blood vessels (these prevent a back flow of blood) are given some rest.

Technique:

1. Lie on your back with a pillow or two under your head and shoulders. Rest your legs against a wall (or other suitable prop). The legs should form about a 45 degree angle with the floor. In positioning yourself, take care not to strain your back. Rest your arms beside you or stretch them out sideways, as preferred.

2. Remain in this position for a few minutes, but not until your feet become cold or numb, or until you feel 'pins and needles' in them. Close your eyes if you wish and maintain a comfortable, rhythmical breathing pattern. In this position you may also, with advantage, practise the Complete Breath, the Breathing Away Fatigue Breath, the Rhythmical Breath, or the Alternate Nostril Breath (section 8). You may also practise the Sponge technique.

Caution:

It is *not* recommended that you have your buttocks close to the wall so that your legs

Fig. 45   *Legs Against the Wall. Legs and floor form a 45° angle.*

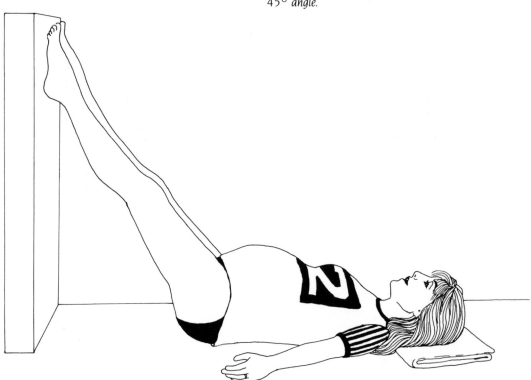

form a right angle with your body. In pregnancy such a position would cause too much pressure on the blood vessels in the groin area.

Meditation

Meditation, according to Dr Lawrence LeShan, author of *How to Meditate* (Aquarian Press, 1983) is doing one thing and only one thing at a time. You focus your attention intently on one object or activity at a time to the exclusion of everything else that's unrelated.

Chief among the benefits derived from regular meditation are deep physiological (referring to body function) relaxation while maintaining alertness of mind; lower metabolic rate; lowered blood pressure — to within normal limits, and increased skin resistance, which indicates decreased anxiety and tension.

Increasingly, doctors are recommending a period of meditation daily for a variety of health disorders. For your own reassurance, however, do *obtain your doctor's permission* to practise the specimen meditation that follows.

Before Meditating

● Choose a quiet place where you are unlikely to be disturbed for ten to twenty minutes.

● Sit comfortably; observe good posture. If necessary, support your head and spine. Relax your facial muscles; pay special attention to your jaws. Relax your hands. Relax the rest of your body. Close your eyes.

● Spend a few moments establishing slow, smooth, natural breathing.

The Meditation

1. Exhale completely through the nostrils.

2. Inhale slowly and smoothly.

3. Exhale and mentally count 'one'.

4. Inhale again.

5. Exhale and mentally count 'two'.

6. Repeat steps 2 to 5, mentally counting 'three' and 'four' with the third and fourth *exhalations*.

7. Repeat steps 2 to 5, again and again in smooth succession, until your predetermined meditation time is up.

8. Open your eyes, leisurely stretch your limbs and/or gently massage any parts of your body that need it, and unhurriedly prepare to resume your usual activities.

Note

As you meditate (especially as a beginner), you may find that your thoughts stray to other matters. Don't be discouraged. It's normal. Simply re-direct your attention to your meditation and begin again. Your perseverance will be worthwhile.

The Breasts

The Chest Expander (modified)

Benefits:

- Strengthens and firms the pectoral muscles supporting the breasts.

- Strengthens and firms the arms.

- Relieves tension and fatigue in the shoulders, which may have resulted from sitting incorrectly at a desk or sewing machine for a long time.

- Contributes to improvement of posture.

- Helps improve chest expansion and ventilation of the lungs.

Technique:

1. Stand with the feet several inches apart and arms at the sides. As a variation, you may sit in one of the sitting postures (section 2), on a stool, or sideways on a chair so as not to have interference from the chair back. Hold the body comfortably erect, and try to minimize the arch of your lower back by tucking in your bottom. Compose yourself.

2. Inhaling, slowly raise the arms sideways until they are at shoulder level. Slowly turn the palms downward.

3. Exhaling, slowly lower the arms to a point

from which you can comfortably swing them behind you in order to clasp the hands together. Feel the shoulderblades

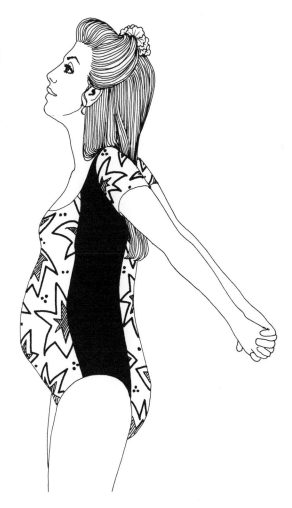

Fig. 46 *Preparing for the Chest Expander (modified).*

119

squeeze together. How good the sensation feels — enjoy it! Now turn the wrists so that the palms of the hands are toward the body.

4. Keeping erect, inhale while you push the still clasped hands upward as far as you comfortably can, keeping the arms straight (Fig. 46). Do this slowly and with control. The tendency, as you push the arms upward, will be to bend forward somewhat. Try to stay upright. Hold the position for a few seconds, breathing normally.

5. Slowly lower the arms as you exhale, unclasp the hands and relax, breathing normally.

Suggestion:

After bending over a desk or sewing machine for, say, half an hour or so, get up and do the Chest Expander. You will be preventing an accumulation of tension in the upper back, and exercising the bust at the same time.

The Head of a Cow Pose (Posture Clasp or Hand Clasp)

Benefits:

● Tones and firms the pectoral muscles.

● Expands the rib cage and improves lung capacity.

● Relieves tension in the shoulders.

Technique:

1. Sit in the Firm Posture (Fig. 15) or another comfortable position.

2. Reach behind your back from below with

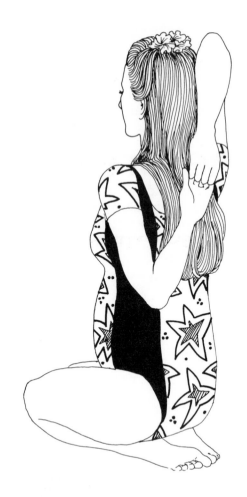

Fig. 47 *Head of a Cow Pose (Posture Clasp or Hand Clasp).*

your left hand, turning the palm away from the body.

3. With the right hand, reach over the right shoulder and try to interlock the fingers of both hands. Impossible? To begin with, you may take a folded scarf in the right hand, throw it over the right shoulder and grasp the free end of it with the left hand. Alternatives to a scarf would be a small, flat cushion held diagonally, a belt or a wash cloth. Keep the body erect and the right elbow pointing straight upward rather than forward. Keep the arm as close to the ear as you can (Fig. 47). Observing these points will help you receive the full benefits of this posture.

4. Hold the position for a few seconds, breathing normally. Keep the fingers firmly interlocked all the time, or if you have used an object to which to hold on, do so securely. If you exert a steady downward pull with the left hand and an upward one with the right hand, you will get the feel of the muscles across the front of the chest working.

5. Unlock the hands (or release the object you have been holding), let the arms fall to the sides of the body, shake the hands a few times and shrug your shoulders. Relax, breathing normally.

6. Repeat the posture, changing the position of the arms, and substituting 'right' for 'left'

and vice versa in the instructions.

Suggestions:

● You are about to zip a dress at the back. When you have reached half way, pause and reach behind you from above with the other hand, interlock the fingers with those of the lower hand, and perform the Head of a Cow pose.

● You are taking a bath and are about to wash your back. Take a few seconds to do the pose just described, with or without the aid of a wash cloth.

Hands to the Wall

Benefits:

● Tones and strengthens a group of muscles which provide power in movements of pushing. The muscles involved are supports of the breasts.

● The wrists and arms are firmed and strengthened.

Technique:

1. Stand erect facing a wall. Place the palms of the hands flat against it. Adjust your stance so that you are at arm's length from the wall. Turn the hands so that the fingers of one point toward those of the other and touch, but do not overlap. Ensure that you are holding yourself well — tuck in your bottom to try to reduce the curve of the small of the back. Keep the shoulders relaxed. Your feet should be firm on the floor, with the body weight equally distributed between them (Fig. 48). Establish an even, comfortable respiration.

2. Maintaining good body alignment, slowly bend the elbows outward as you begin to

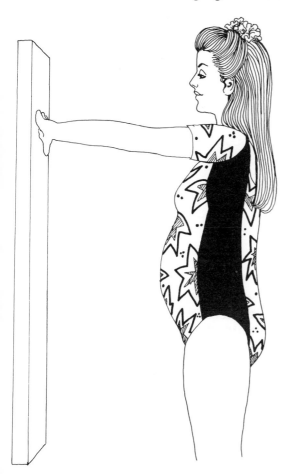

Fig. 48 Preparing for the Hands to the Wall pose.

121

3. When your face is as near to the wall as you can manage with comfort, hold the position for a few seconds, breathing normally.

4. Slowly reverse the movement while inhaling. Use the same slow, controlled action of resistance as you push yourself away from the wall. Relax, breathing normally.

Bust Exercise (The Palm Press)

Benefits:

● Tones and strengthens the pectoral muscles supporting the breasts.

● Improves the blood supply to the tissues underlying the breasts.

● Helps release tension from the hands.

● It is believed that regular performance of this exercise can contribute to enhancing lactation.

Technique:

1. Sit comfortably in one of the sitting postures (section 2), on a chair or stool. You may also stand.

2. Inhaling, bring the arms sideways to shoulder level, then bend and move them inward across the front of the chest, placing the hands together in front of the sternum (breast-bone) in the namaste or prayer position (Fig. 50). Note the alignment of the forearms from elbow to elbow.

3. Exhale. Now establish a comfortable breathing pattern, deeply inhaling and exhaling in a slow, smooth and even fashion. This pattern established, press the two palms firmly together, exerting a steady pressure with on palm against the opposing palm. This is an isometric-type

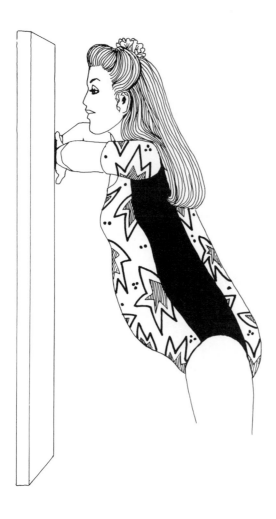

Fig. 49 *The completed Hands to the Wall pose.*

push against the wall in a steady and controlled manner, gradually bringing the face toward it (Fig. 49). The movement should be one of firm, steady resistance. In this way the muscles of the arms and chest will receive the utmost benefit. Do this forward motion while exhaling. Keep the body as a straight line; do not bend at the knees or waist. Let your arms do the work.

exercise which appears to be more effective than alternately pressing together and releasing the palms a number of times. You should feel the muscles across the front of the chest working as you press the palms together and maintain the pressure. Breathe normally as you hold the position, then release after a few seconds and relax.

Notes:

- Namaste is an Indian gesture implying respect. It is used, for example, when greeting someone.
- The Blade (see section 6) is another posture of value in firming the bustline.

Suggestion:

The foregoing exercise may be done at a convenient moment while watching television or waiting for the tea kettle to boil.

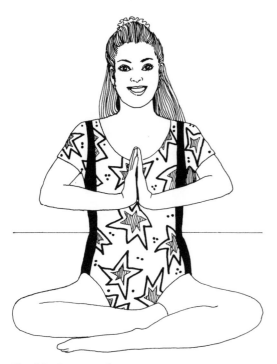

Fig. 50 *Preparing for a Bust Exercise — the Namaste or Prayer position.*

The Respiratory System and Breathing

The Complete Breath

Technique:

1. Choose a comfortable position. It may be sitting, standing or lying. Ensure that the spine is naturally erect (if lying it should be held to its maximum length without strain). There should be no exaggeration of the arch at the lower back, and the body, including the facial muscles, should be relaxed.

2. Following an exhalation, place the hands lightly on the abdomen just below the ribs, with the fingers of one hand touching those of the other (Fig. 51). Keep the shoulders relaxed. Try not to tense the hands and fingers.

3. Slowly inhale, allowing the air to pass toward the back of the throat (pharynx) as it enters the lungs. As the bottom of the lungs fill, you should be aware of a gentle upward rising of the abdomen. This may be

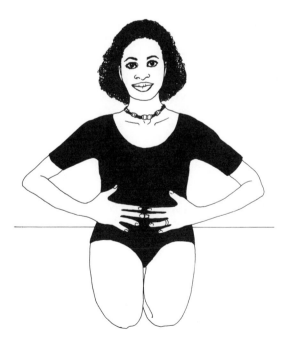

Fig. 51   The Complete Breath — exhalation phase. The ribcage is relaxed.

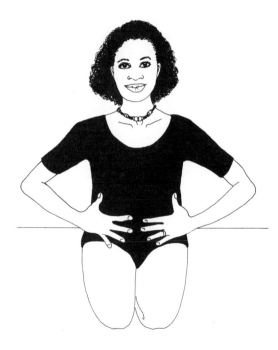

Fig. 52   The Complete Breath — inhalation phase. The ribcage expands.

125

the opposite of your usual mode of breathing, but it is the correct one. Confused? Memorize the following: A*ir in, abdomen out; air out, abdomen in.* Continue inhaling smoothly, filling the middle of the lungs. Note the separation of the fingers as the rib cage expands (Fig. 52). Complete the inhalation until the lungs are filled to capacity without the least feeling of straining. As the inhalation reaches completion, you will sense a slight contraction of the upper abdomen.

4. Now, without holding the breath begin to exhale slowly and smoothly, completely emptying the lungs of stale air. As the exhalation ends, you will feel the abdominal muscles contract, and the fingers will again touch in midline (Fig. 51).

5. Following exhalation, there will be a brief, natural pause prior to the urge to inhale. On feeling this urge inhale as before, and continue breathing as outlined for half a minute or so, to begin with. Gradually increase the length of time you breathe in this fashion. In due course, the length of both inhalation and exhalation will also be greater.

Notes:

● If your abdomen is already quite large, you may find that by placing the hands over the sides of your lower rib cage, you can better sense the rhythmical expansion and contraction of the lungs. The rib cage will move outward on inhalation and inward on exhalation, like an accordion.

● If you have a small child, say under five or so years of age, wait until he or she is sleeping and observe his or her breathing. Note the rhythmic rise and fall of the abdomen, with little movement of the upper chest. This is the natural way to breathe!

The Alternate Nostril Breath

General:

There are several interpretations of the way in which this type of breathing works. One is that the energy which flows through the right nostril during inhalation is catabolic (referring to the breakdown of cells), whereas that flowing through the left nostril is anabolic (building up). These two processes, building up and breaking down, constitute metabolism. In practising alternate nostril breathing, you are endeavouring to establish harmony between the two processes. If this harmony is achieved, it manifests itself in a calmer state of mind and better emotional balance. Emotional instability in pregnancy is not uncommon.

Benefits:

● Soothes the nervous system. Practise it whenever you feel tension or anxiety mounting, depression or frustration setting in. Practise it before making a public appearance, if you feel nervous.

● A natural sedative. Practised at bedtime, it can help overcome insomnia.

● Helps keep the blood pressure within normal limits.

Technique:

1. Sit or lie in a comfortable position. Posture should be correct.

2. Relax the left hand and arm. Raise the right arm and arrange the fingers as depicted in Figure 53. As an alternative to curling the middle two fingers toward the palm of the hand, you may rest them lightly on the forehead, above the bridge of the nose. Keep the hand and fingers as relaxed as you can. You may close your eyes for better concentration and to promote rest.

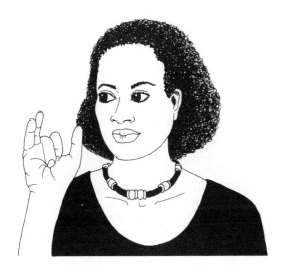

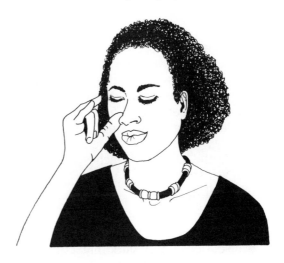

Fig. 53 *Preparing for Alternate Nostril breathing. Note the arrangement of the fingers of the right hand.*

Fig. 54 *The Alternate Nostril Breath. The right thumb is used to close the right nostril.*

3. Placing the right thumb gently against the right nostril, close it (Fig. 54), exhaling slowly, smoothly, and completely through the left nostril. Let the air pass toward the back of the throat.

4. Follow exhalation by a smooth, even inhalation through the left nostril, maintaining closure of the right nostril. Let the inflow of air be directed toward the back of

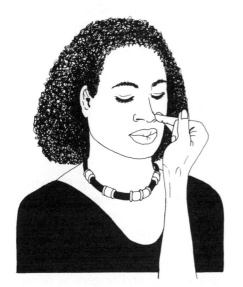

Fig. 55 *The Alternate Nostril Breath. The right ring finger is used to close the left nostril.*

the throat, and try to keep the breath inaudible.

5. Inhalation completed, proceed *without* retaining the breath to release closure of the right nostril while simultaneously closing the left nostril with the ring finger, or ring and little fingers (Fig. 55). Exhale through the right nostril slowly, effortlessly and thoroughly.

6. Exhalation is then followed by another smoothly flowing inhalation, again through the right nostril.

7. The right nostril is closed by the right thumb, the finger (or fingers) removed from the left nostril through which a slow, complete exhalation takes place to finalize one round of alternate nostril breathing.

8. Lower the hand and relax, breathing normally.

9. Repeat steps 2 to 8 one or more times. You need not pause between rounds; you may instead do a chosen number of rounds and then resume your normal breathing.

Notes:

- Your partner or a friend can read the instructions to you at the beginning, until you know the pattern by heart. If your helper is your partner, here is yet another opportunity to involve him in your pregnancy.

- Usually, the length of the inhalation is in a certain ratio to that of the exhalation, but this varies with the individual. For example, you may inhale for a count of four and exhale for a count of six. If you wish to time your respirations (this gives you something else on which to focus), make quite sure that you are absolutely comfortable with your chosen number of counts. No strain whatever should be involved.

The Rhythmic Breath

Benefits:

- Gives energy.

- Soothes the nervous system.

- Helps restore emotional balance.

Technique:

1. Sit or lie comfortably. You may also do this breath while walking. Maintain good posture. Close your eyes if you wish, and keep the body relaxed.

2. Decide on a method of timing your respirations. Here are a few suggestions:

- Mentally count 'Om 1, Om 2, Om 3', etc., or, 'one hundred, two hundred, three hundred', etc. (om is a Sanskrit word symbolic of the whole range of creation)

- Imagine yourself to be hearing slow, measured footsteps on the sidewalk; count them: one and two and three, etc.

- Mentally beat time to a suitable piece of

imagined music. It should be of slow, even tempo.
(Whatever your method of timing, the beats must be slow and of equal duration.)

3. Begin respiration by exhaling completely, feeling your abdomen tighten as you do so.

4. Inhale deeply, slowly, smoothly and regularly in accordance with the counting pattern you have predetermined. Adhere strictly to this rhythm throughout.

5. Without pausing, exhale in the same manner.

6. Repeat the cycle — inhalation followed by exhalation in a smoothly flowing current. Practise this rhythmical breathing for half a minute or so, to begin with.

Caution:

It is not a good idea to use the pulse beat as a device for marking time at a desired rate. You see, at the very times the Rhythmic Breath would be indicated, such as in states of anxiety and excitement, the pulse rate is inclined to be rapid and sometimes irregular. To match the breathing to such a rate and rhythm would be undesirable. What we want is a slow, regular breath so as to effect a corresponding evenness of the emotions.

Note:

When breathing in this way it is almost impossible to panic. Whenever you feel the onset of apprehension, fear, irritability, anxiety, frustration or anger, practise rhythmic breathing to restore mental and emotional balance. Use it also for the relief of minor aches and pains. It will sometimes ease pressure which may be causing such discomforts, as well as focus attention away from the discomforts themselves.

The Walking Breath

Practise this breath for part of your walk out of doors.

Benefits:

- Revitalizes the body.
- Calms the nerves.

Technique:

1. Ensure that your body is erect and comfortable. Buttocks should be tucked in, reducing the arch of the lower back. Shoulders should be relaxed and shoulderblades back. Exhale completely.

2. Slowly inhale for the duration of three, four or more steps, as best suits you, thus: Inhale 1 step, 2 steps, 3 steps, (4 steps or more).

3. Without pausing, exhale 1 step, 2 steps, 3 steps, (4 steps or more).

4. Repeat 2 and 3 for a total of twenty or thirty seconds, to begin with, increasing the length of time as your breathing improves.

Note:

Practise this breath for only a small part of your walk to begin with, so as to allow your lungs time to accommodate to what is perhaps an unaccustomed intake of oxygen all at once. If you suddenly take in too much oxygen, the lungs become overventilated (hyperventilation), and you may experience dizziness. As your breathing apparatus becomes stronger, you will find that you can comfortably increase the number of steps you take with both inhalation and exhalation. Try to make exhalation a little longer than inhalation, to ensure thorough emptying of the lungs.

'Breathing Away Fatigue' Breath

Benefits:

- Relaxes and refreshes body and mind.

Technique:

1. Lie or sit comfortably. If you wish, elevate your legs by resting them against a piece of furniture or a wall (Fig. 45, p.116). Legs and floor should form about a 45 degree angle. Close your eyes, Relax the body. Relax the facial muscles.

2. Exhale thoroughly.

3. Inhale slowly, deeply and smoothly, allowing the air to flow toward the back of the throat. Visualize this air flow as, perhaps, a cool, soothing beam of light which brings to the body energy, lightness and balance. Imagine the air filled with life-giving prana and oxygen, revitalizing every body cell.

4. Inhalation completed, proceed without pause to exhale slowly, smoothly and completely, visualizing as you do so an outflow of fatigue poisons, aches, pains, heaviness and all negative feelings, in one irreversible stream.

5. Continue breathing in this manner until you feel totally refreshed, relaxed and revitalized.

Caution:

If you have chosen to lie with your legs elevated, do not keep them in this position for too long — certainly not until you experience cold or numbness in the legs. Make sure also that there is no pressure on the calf muscles, if you are resting them on a piece of furniture. If you are near a wall, the buttocks should not be touching it, because in this position there would be compression of the large blood vessels in the groin area. Adjust the bottom so that it is far enough from the wall so that when you rest the legs against it, they form a 45-degree angle with the floor.

The Mountain Posture

Benefits:

- Tones the nervous system.

- Expands the rib cage fully, allowing for a better intake of oxygen and improved lung capacity.

- Tones and strengthens the muscles of the entire trunk: chest, abdomen and pelvis.

- Helps digestion and improves elimination.

- Promotes general relaxation.

- Helps flatten the abdomen, postnatally, by throwing the abdominal organs firmly backward and upward against the spine. Pressure on the pelvic organs is reduced.

- Helps strengthen pelvic structures and discourages uterine prolapse.

Technique:

1. Sit comfortably in one of the cross-legged positions, trunk naturally erect, shoulders and facial muscles relaxed. As an alternative sitting position you may use the Firm Posture (Fig. 15), or you may sit on a chair.

2. Place the hands in front of, but not touching the chest, in the prayer (or namaste) position.

3. Exhale completely. Keeping the palms pressed together, inhale while slowly raising the arms above the head until you have reached your ultimate comfortable stretch (Fig. 56). The upper arms should be alongside the ears, and chin should not be jutting forward. You would invite tension in the lower jaw and neck by so doing. Eyes can be focused on a chosen spot or object in front of you to help you concentrate better. Relax your facial muscles.

4. Hold the position for a few seconds, breathing slowly and rhythmically.

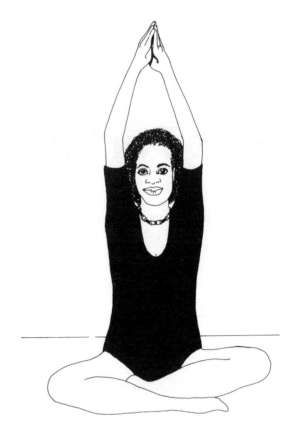

Fig. 56   The Mountain Posture.

5. Slowly lower the arms as you exhale, bringing them, palms still pressed together, in front of your chest.

6. Relax the arms, resting the hands quietly in the lap or on the knees. Relax the whole body, breathing normally.

7. Repeat once or twice.

Note:

Be reassured that there is no truth in the 'old wives' tale' that stretching upward during pregnancy can cause the umbilical cord to injure the foetus. You must, however, remember to stretch only to your comfortable limit.

Post Partum

Reminder: Please refer to chapter 13 (Post Partum). It is very important to *check with your doctor* before starting on any exercise regimen.

Prone Relaxation Posture

Benefits:

- Helps flatten the abdomen more quickly.

- Assists the uterus in returning to its normal position.

- Contributes to complete physical and mental relaxation.

Technique:

1. Lie prone (face downward), body stretched out at full length, limbs relaxed.

2. The toes should point toward each other and the heels fall apart.

3. Arms should lie passively on either side of the body or folded above the head; the face is turned to one side. Change the direction to which your face is turned after a while or the next time you lie in this position.

4. Either place a pillow under your head or make a 'pillow' of your arms and rest your head on this.

5. Place one or two pillows under the hips and abdomen. This will reduce the arch at the small of the back and prevent strain on the back muscles.

6. Your breasts should fall freely between the two sets of pillows and not be compressed. Compression may cause pain, especially if

Fig. 57 Prone Relaxation Posture. Cushions are used to enhance relaxation.

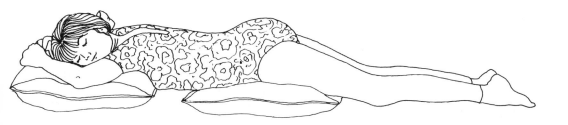

131

you are nursing. (Position depicted in Fig. 57).

7. Follow the same relaxation technique as in the Sponge (section 6).

Note:

Use this position, especially during the first few days post partum, when having your afternoon nap.

Caution:

Lying prone without some support under the hips is not recommended. It would accentuate the curve of the spine at the lower back, and place strain on the muscles and ligaments in that area.

Leg Over

Benefits:

● Firms and strengthens the oblique and transverse abdominal muscles and those of the lower back.

● Trims the waist line.

● Tones and helps slenderize the areas along the inner thighs.

Technique:

1. Lie on your back with legs together and outstretched. Position your arms so they are pointing sideways, at shoulder level. Your body and limbs should resemble a letter 'T'. Keep your back pressed firmly to the surface on which you are lying.

2. Raise the left leg slowly upward and then across the body to touch the floor on your right side. Do this either on exhalation or inhalation. Simultaneously turn the head to the left, keeping the hands, arms and shoulders in contact with the floor (Fig. 58).

3. Hold for a second or two, breathing normally. Combining suitable breathing, slowly bring the left leg up and lower it to the floor in front of you.

4. Relax, breathing normally. Repeat steps 2 and 3, this time raising the right leg and turning the head to the right. (Substitute 'right' for 'left', and vice versa, in the instructions.)

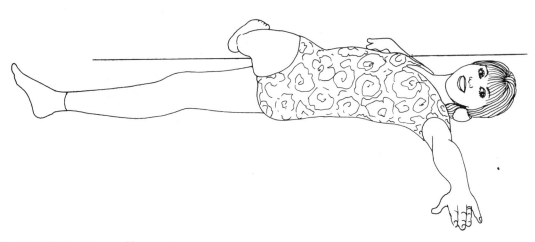

Fig. 58 The Leg Over position.

Note:

The Leg Over is more effective if the hands, arms and shoulders are kept in contact with the floor, even if you cannot lower the leg as much as you would wish. If necessary, hold onto a stable piece of furniture, to begin with.

The Pelvic Twist

Benefits:

● Firms and strengthens the oblique and transverse abdominal muscles and those of the lower back.

● Trims the waist line.

Technique:

1. Lie on your back with legs together and outstretched. Position your arms so they are pointing sideways, at shoulder level.

2. Bend the legs at the knees and, exhaling, draw them toward the chest.

3. Inhaling, lower the knees to the floor on your right side while simultaneously turning your head to the left. The hands, arms and shoulders should remain in contact with the floor (Fig. 59).

4. Hold for a second or two, then slowly and carefully bring the legs up to the chest as you exhale, and lower them to the floor in front of you as you inhale. Relax, breathing normally.

5. Repeat steps 2 to 4, lowering the legs to the left and turning the head to the right this time. (Substitute 'left' for 'right', and vice versa, in the instructions.)

Variation:

1. From the position described in step 1 of the Technique, bend the legs just enough to enable you to place the soles of the feet flat on the floor.

2. Keeping the hands, arms and shoulders anchored, let the knees fall towards the floor on your right as you turn your head to the left.

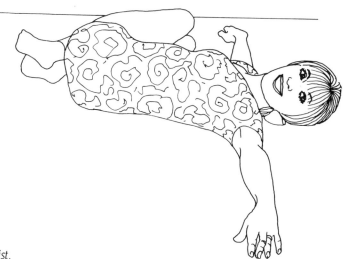

Fig. 59 The Pelvic Twist.

3. Repeat to the other side. Combine suitable breathing.

The Cat Stretch

Caution: It is very important to *check with your doctor* before practising the following exercise sequence. Step 2 (Fig. 61), done earlier than six weeks following the birth of your baby, poses risks of air emboli (air bubbles in the blood vessels or chambers of the heart).

Benefits:

● Tones and strengthens the muscles of the back and abdomen.

● Helps keep the spine supple.

● Assists the uterus in returning to its normal position.

● Improves the pelvic blood circulation. During pregnancy the weight of the uterus had compressed pelvic blood vessels, slowing down the circulation.

● Helps relieve backache.

Technique:

1. With arms and legs comfortably apart, adopt an 'all fours' position on hands and knees. Thighs and arms should be roughly perpendicular to the trunk (Fig. 60).

2. Inhaling, bend your elbows and attempt to lower the chest to the floor (Fig. 61). Thighs should remain perpendicular to the body, and back should not be allowed to sag. Keep the head bent slightly backward so that the neck receives a delightful stretch as the chin also touches the floor. Let the hands and arms take most of the weight so

Fig. 60   Preparing for the Cat Stretch — the 'all fours' position.

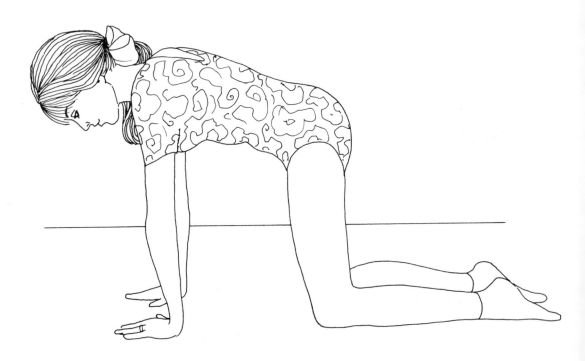

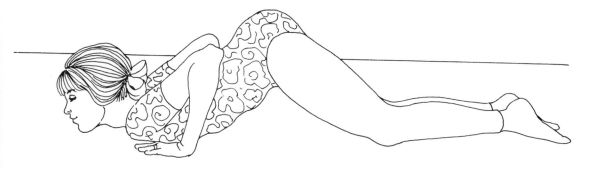

Fig. 61 *The Cat Stretch — the 'Knee-chest' position.*

that no undesirable pressure is exerted on the lower back.

3. Hold the position for several seconds, breathing normally.

4. Exhaling, return to the starting position described in step 1 (Fig. 60). Remain thus for a few seconds, breathing normally.

5. Exhaling, lower your head, hunch your back and bring your left knee toward your forehead (Fig. 62). Hold the position for a second or two.

6. Inhaling, push the leg backward and

Fig. 62 *The Cat Stretch — the 'Knee-to-forehead' position.*

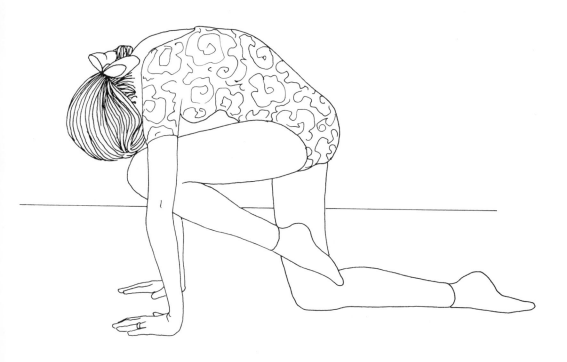

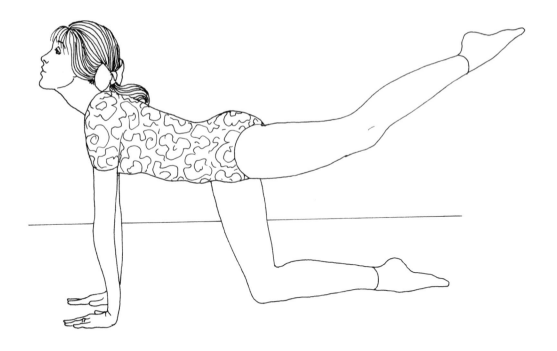

Fig. 63   *The Cat Stretch — an all-body stretch.*

stretch it upward as far as you can, while bringing the head upward and backward (Fig. 63). Keep the leg as straight as possible. Hold for a second or two, breathing normally.

7. Exhaling, lower the knee to the floor and relax for a few seconds, breathing normally. Relax the neck.

8. Repeat steps 5 to 7, using the right leg this time.

9. Lie down and relax, breathing slowly and rhythmically.

Notes:

Step 2 describes what is known in medical circles as the 'knee-chest' position. When this position is held, the pressure of abdominal viscera on pelvic organs is relieved, and the uterus gravitates forward into its normal position. In addition to being used as part of the Cat Stretch series, this pose may be used as a complete asana in itself. Practised daily, it will help the uterus return to its prepregnant position speedily.

Please refer to the *caution* on page 134 preceding the instructions for this exercise sequence.

Adjust the position of the arms and hands for maximum comfort (try turning the hands so that the fingers point toward each other). Remember not to exert too much downward pressure on the small of the back, and make sure that the bladder is empty before you begin practice.

The 'knee-chest' position is useful in helping correct retroversion (tipping backward) of the uterus. It is a fairly common condition following repeated childbearing, and may be due to excessive relaxation of some pelvic structures. Signs and symptoms of this condition include backache and persistent vaginal discharge.

Side Leg Raise (One-Legged Lateral Posture)

Benefits:

● Trims the waist line.

● Reduces fatty deposits from the inner thighs.

● Tones the pelvic floor.

Technique:

1. Lie on your right side, supporting the head with your right hand. Place the palm of the left hand on the floor in front of you for stability and balance. You may bend the right leg slightly. Ideally, the body from right armpit to knee should be in alignment.

2. Inhaling, slowly raise the left leg upward, keeping it directly over the right one rather than behind or in front of it. Try to hold the raised leg as straight as possible (Fig. 64).

3. Hold the position for a second or two, breathing as normally as you can.

4. Exhaling, slowly lower the leg. Relax, breathing normally.

5. Repeats steps 1 to 4, substituting 'left' for 'right' and vice versa in the instructions.

Fig. 64 The Side Leg Raise (One-legged Lateral Posture).

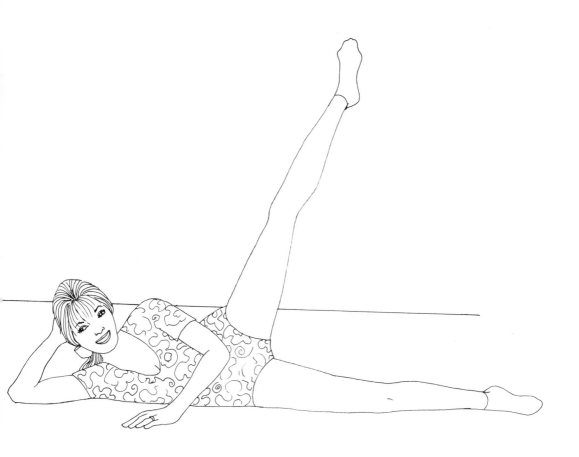

Glossary
of Technical Terms

Adductor muscle
Any muscle which draws a limb toward the mid-line of the body.

Aeration
Supplying with air.

Anatomical
Referring to the structure of the body.

Anaemia
Deficiency in quality or quantity of the red blood cells.

Anus
Outlet of the rectum (lower end of large intestine).

Asanas
Poses, postures, or exercises.

Breech
Presentation of the foetus when the buttocks and/or the feet are closest to the cervix (neck of womb) and will be born before the head.

Coccyx
'Tail-bone'. The last bone at the bottom of the spine. It is formed by four small bones which are fused.

Diaphragm
Large dome-shaped muscle separating the chest from the abdomen; important muscle of respiration (breathing process).

Episiotomy
Surgical incision of perineal body (of which perineum is external surface) to make birth smoother, to prevent laceration, and avoid damage to head of baby.

Foetus
Describes the unborn child from the third month to the end of pregnancy.

Haemorrhoids
Piles. Dilated and sometimes inflamed veins of the rectum.

Hatha Yoga
System of physical exercises, breathing techniques and hygiene practices.

Intercostal
Between the ribs. Intercostal muscles are muscles of the chest wall.

Intervertebral discs
Thin pads of cartilage between the vertebrae (bones) forming the spine.

Intrauterine
Within the uterus.

Isometric
Brief tensing of a muscle.

Involution
Describes the rapid decrease in size of the uterus after childbirth.

Lactation
Secretion of nourishment from the breasts for the baby.

Levator ani muscle
Muscle which helps the anus contract. One of the supports of the pelvic organs.

Ligament
Fibrous tissue connecting bones which form a joint.

Lumbar
Refers to the small of the back between the ribs and the hip bones.

Miscarriage
Expulsion of the foetus before the end of the seventh month of pregnancy.

Neuromuscular
Refers to nerves and muscles.

Oxygenate
To saturate with oxygen.

Pectoral muscles
Muscles of the chest.

Perineum
The tissues between the anus and external genitals.

Physiological
Refers to the functions of the body.

Piles
See haemorrhoids.

Placenta
Afterbirth. Organ made up of many vessels, which supplies the unborn baby with nourishment through the umbilical cord.

Postnatal
After birth.

Prenatal
Before birth.

Prolapse
Falling downward.

Prone
Lying face downward.

Psychoprophylaxis
From Greek 'psyche', mind, and 'prophylactikos', guarding. Describes a method of mental and physical preparation for natural childbirth.

Pubic
Refers to the external genitals.

Rectum
End of the large intestine.

Sacroiliac
Refers to the joints where the top part of the hip bones meet the lower part of the spine, roughly just above the buttocks.

Sacrum
A triangular bone forming the back of the pelvis.

Skeletal
Refers to the bony framework of the body.

Sphincter
A ring-like muscle which, when contracted, closes an orifice, e.g. the anus.

Stress incontinence of urine
Inability to retain urine when coughing, sneezing, jumping, etc.

Supine
Lying on the back with the face upward.

Umbilical cord
The connection through which the unborn baby receives nourishment from the mother.

Urethra
A narrow canal through which urine is discharged from the bladder.

Uterus
Womb.

Vagina
Muscular canal leading from the uterus to the external genitals.

Varicose veins
Swollen veins, usually of the legs.

Viscera
The organs of the body's cavities. Usually refers to the intestines.

Index